MENTAL HEALTH MAKEOVER:
THE 5-STEP PLAN FOR TAKING CHARGE OF YOUR DIAGNOSIS AND LIVING A HAPPY, BALANCED LIFE

by

Laura E. Gray, Ph.D.

Copyright 2019

Dedication

Dedication and Acknowledgments

This book is dedicated to my immediate family: to my husband, Brian; my sons Corey and Hunter; and my daughter Logan. In addition, I want to send a special thanks to my mom, Barbara, who has always believed in me and knew I had something to offer in spite of my mental illness.

I'd like to thank the following people, also, who have helped me tremendously along the way: to Beth C and Alfonso G, the two best therapists EVER; Aaron Z and Alonso M, the best psychiatric nurse practitioner and the psychiatrist I know; Paulette G, my very good friend and family doctor; Tracy M, my BFF; and Jennifer M and Melissa C, my other partners in crime.

I know there are countless others out there who have done more for me than I could ever repay them for, but I'd probably end up writing another 2000 words if I tried to name them all.

To all of you: thank you for loving me and helping to shape my journey. It's been incredible.

Introduction

Thank you for picking up this book. I should probably be the first to tell you that this is no ordinary "how to get well in 30 days" kind of book. In fact, I'm not going to tell you how to get well. I'm not even going to tell you which medicines you should be taking or why you were diagnosed with whatever you were diagnosed with in the first place. The truth is—I don't know why you and I were diagnosed with our illnesses, and I'm certainly no expert on psychotropic medications, not having even heard of some of the newer ones.

What I am going to tell you, though, is that you don't have to be just "okay." You don't have to just survive. Believe it or not, you can live the life you always wanted—the life of your dreams, even—by following the five simple steps I've outlined in this book. Will it be easy? Probably not. (Remember I said the steps were simple, not easy.) But I can guarantee you that it will be rewarding in the end, and you will probably end up being glad you read the book.

I'm just an ordinary person who was diagnosed with an ordinary mental illness (two, actually) a long time ago. And for the first eighteen years after being diagnosed, I didn't follow these five steps, and I didn't feel very good for more than a month or two at a time. What I'm trying to say is this: If I can do this, so can you. So can anybody. We deserve so much more than to just be "okay." And we have the power within ourselves—with a little help from our medical community, family, and friends—to be fantastic!

Enjoy the read!

~Laura

CHAPTER 1

Mid-Life Crisis in the Extreme

Something happened to me when I turned thirty-five. All of a sudden I didn't feel "young" anymore. I didn't exactly feel middle-aged, but the feeling of being young and carefree had left me. It wasn't as if I had exactly been carefree for the last ten or twelve years, either. I had married my first husband at 23 and divorced him at 24 and remarried again at 25 in what was kind of a self-imposed shotgun wedding to a guy who was by no means ready to take on the responsibility of marriage or kids, gotten pregnant (not necessarily in that order), had a miscarriage at 13 weeks, gotten pregnant again six months later, and had a baby at the age of twenty-six. And oh yeah—did I mention that this marriage was even worse than the first?

By 30 I had had a second child with husband number two, divorced husband number two (again, not necessarily in that order), lost a home, filed bankruptcy, gotten my master's degree, and had a career change, met the REAL man of my dreams, married said man of my dreams, had two more miscarriages, had a high-risk pregnancy, gave birth to child number three, and bought a second home.

So why, again, had I felt young in the first place before my 35th birthday? Maybe it was because up until that point, I hadn't found any gray hairs on my head. Or maybe it was because my gynecologist hadn't recommended that I get off the pill because I was getting too "old" to be on it. Heck, I don't know. Maybe I just didn't think about my age before then. But there was something about turning 35 that bothered me that hadn't bothered me on any of my previous birthdays. The day I turned 35, it dawned on me that I was on the downside to 40, and 40 was OFFICIALLY MIDDLE AGE!

So… what does Middle Age look like? I think it can look different, depending on who you are. If you're a guy, I don't think it's a lot different than any other age. I mean, I know there's the stereotype of men who go through the typical midlife crisis. They color their gray hair or get hair plugs or a bad hairpiece to cover up the bald spots. They might go out and buy a sports car or flashy jewelry, and the worst of them have an affair, or if they're divorced, they start dating women half their age. Anything to feel young again, right?

But for women it's different. And for women who have a history of depression, anxiety, or any other mental health issue, it's vastly different. Here's what it looked like for me:

I had been diagnosed with Bipolar Disorder at the age of 21, but other than popping a few pills every day, seeing my psychiatrist every so often, and visiting a psychologist when things were going wrong—which was more often than I wanted to admit—I pretty much denied that there was a problem. I didn't answer "yes" on job applications when asked if I had a disability or a history of psychiatric problems (which was pretty ironic since I was working as a school counselor at the time), I didn't let even people who were very close to me know my mental health history, and I walked around and acted as if I were the most normal person in the world.

Of course, that strategy, if you can call it that, tended to backfire on a regular basis. By my 36th birthday, I had had to go to inpatient hospitalization no less than three times in the last two years, once for a profoundly serious suicide attempt. Not cool at all. Of course, I had gone back to work as if nothing had happened at all, even though I'm positive that many people knew exactly what had happened.

In addition to being in acute denial over my mental health issues, I was juggling WAY too much. I was about 2/3 of the way through a doctoral program where I was taking anywhere from two to three courses a semester, some online and some at the university, which was a full 70 miles from my home. I had three children, two of whom were in elementary school and one who was in preschool. And oh, by the way, all three had been diagnosed with ADHD, and one had Asperger's Syndrome. My husband worked long hours away from home. I was working full-time at a job I really didn't like. So, you know, it's not as if I had a lot on my plate or anything, being the over-achiever that I was (and still am).

Of course, on the outside and to the outside world, everything probably looked fine. We had a nice home in a middle-class neighborhood. Our kids were doing well, and they were happy. Our middle son was an all-star baseball player who played for a travel team and whom my husband coached on his regular season little league team. Our older son had had some issues but was doing very well in school. Our daughter was cute and wore adorable clothes that her grandmother made and monogrammed for her. I had been the organist and choir director at our church for umpteen years and had worked in the public school system in the same town where I had grown up. What could possibly be abnormal about all of that, right?

To put it bluntly, I was incredibly overwhelmed and just wasn't happy—not at work, not in school, not with myself, not about much of anything. So I hit my mid-thirties, and it was like, "What in the hell am I doing, how the hell did it get to this, and what the hell do I do about it now???"

I bet you're not really surprised to hear that, are you? The truth is, many, many people—women in particular—the overwhelming majority, in fact, somewhere between the ages of 35 and 55, reach a point in their lives (sometimes more than one, but more about that later) where they stop and say,

"Woah! How did it get to THIS, and what on earth do I do NOW?"

And for those of us who have a history of mental illness or mental health issues, we are almost guaranteed to reach that point at least once during those years. There are several reasons for that. One is due to hormones and simple (ha!) aging. As we age, our hormones are changing, and as you know, the older we get, the less estrogen we produce, until Bam! One day we reach menopause. But don't worry—this is NOT a book about menopause. I positively LOATHE all the doom and gloom books and websites out there about "surviving" menopause and how we all need to just meditate and do yoga to get past the hot flashes and mood swings and hold hands and sing Kum Ba Ya and embrace our womanhood together. Yuck! Nope, you're not going to find that here. But I digress…

Anyway, part of the that is aging and hormones and all that. As our estrogen starts to deplete, our moods shift, and this affects us, especially when we have a history of depression, anxiety, and the like. Men tend to experience drops in testosterone, too, which can affect them just as badly. So there's that. And then there's the whole stage-of-life thing. If we have children, they're getting older, maybe high school-aged or graduating from high school and heading to college. You know—the whole empty nest thing. And children aside, we get to a point in our careers around that time where we've either gotten as far as we can go or we realize that this is NOT what we want to be doing until we retire (that's what happened to me). And if you're married, maybe you've reached a point of stagnation after this time or things are just "different" now that the kids are gone or are about to be gone. So yeah, lots and lots of changes on top of the hormone stuff on top of the depression, anxiety, etc. No wonder we wake up one day and say What The Fuck?!?!?

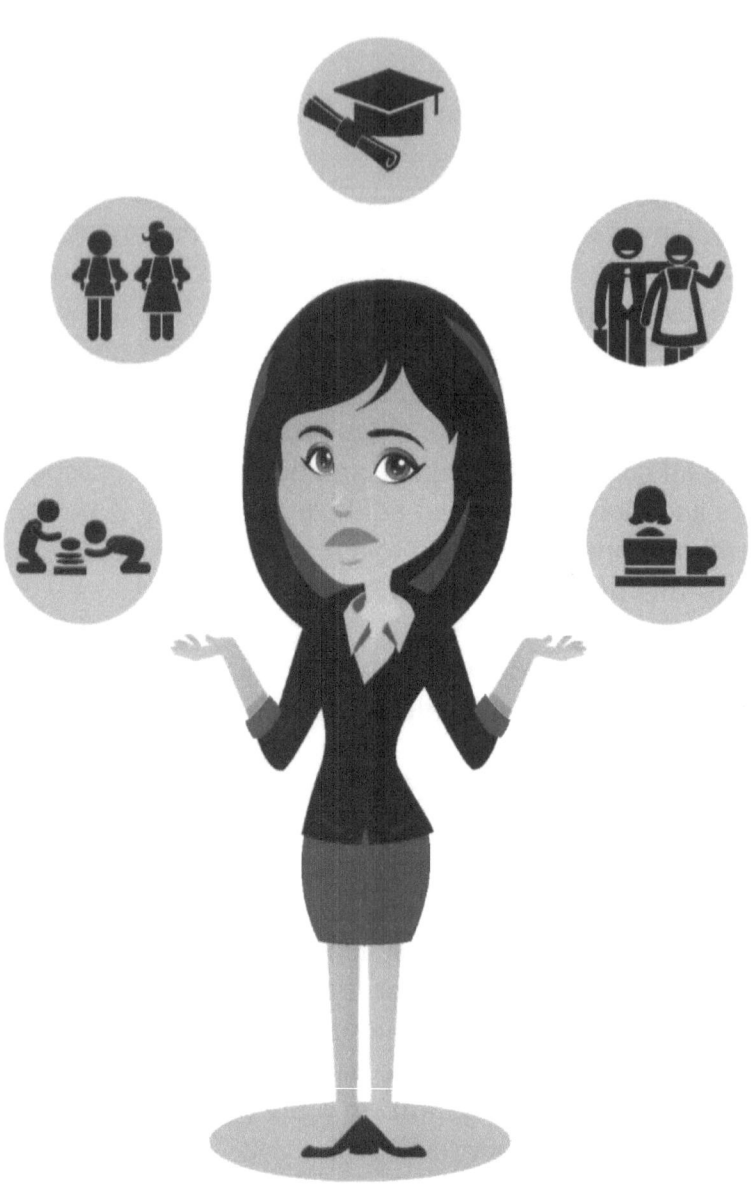

CHAPTER 2

The Epiphany

Now that I've painted a picture of my life—complete with a history of mental health issues, let me tell you that it doesn't ALL have to be doom and gloom. After the "crisis", living with a mental illness doesn't have to be so bad.

So let me tell you about my crisis at 36 and the epiphany that happened when I was 39.

Let's go back to me at 36. Unhappy. Unsatisfied with my life. And downright depressed. I mean, very, very depressed. It was late October, and I was completely overwhelmed. For some reason, Octobers have never been very good for me. My parents split up in October of 1983, I was diagnosed with Bipolar Disorder after a nasty suicide attempt in October of 1991, my last suicide attempt was in October of 2004, and here it was October again. We were all asleep on a Monday night, very late, when my husband got a call from his sister. My mother-in-law had had a massive brain bleed and was in the hospital about to undergo brain surgery to remove the clot. Not good. So my husband hurriedly got up, got dressed, and got on the road. I was at home with the 3 kids.

He was gone for the next couple of days to see about his mom, and I got the kids up and dressed for school each day, which seemed like a positively Herculean task. That Friday, he had to go back to see about his mother, so he left super early in the morning, and when I went to wake the kids, I stopped in the front bathroom to see that the medicine cabinet was open and a large bottle of Prozac had been opened and was spilled all over the counter. There was a trail of pills leading to our four-year old daughter's room, where she was fast asleep. On her floor was a black Sharpie, and pictures were drawn all over her yellow painted walls.

I ignored the drawings and quickly woke her up, asking how many pills she had eaten. She said two, but I really had no way of knowing. I called my mom, got the boys up and dressed, and called my school to tell my principal I needed to take my daughter to the emergency room. Of course, he wasn't happy. He was never happy when I missed a day when the kids were sick. Evidently his children had never been ill a day in their lives, or he had had the luxury of having a close relative to watch them when they were. At any rate, he just did not understand when parents had to stay home with sick kids. Lovely.

So I took Daughter Dearest to the ER, where they treated her with Ipecac, and we spent the day at home while the boys were at school. Of course, this added to my feelings of stress and depression. I remember nothing about the weekend. Not a thing. On Monday, my husband went back to the north part of the state to visit his mom in the hospital, as she had a long road ahead of her in terms of recovery and rehabilitation, and we still didn't know what kind of damage there would be or if she would fully recover from the bleed (I'm happy to say she made a full recovery). I got the kids ready and went to work, as usual.

Then at about 1:00 in the afternoon, a wave washed over me that I still can't explain. I started crying and couldn't stop. I went to the school nurse's office and told her, "I can't do this anymore. I can't stay here." I think she knew what I meant. Luckily, my principal was off campus. Looking back, there's no way he would have understood what was going on, so that was a blessing. The nurse called my mom, and that was my last day to work at that school. I cried all the way home. I knew at that point that I could not work there anymore. I also knew that my days as a doctoral student were over (at least for the next five years or so). I couldn't do anything anymore. I guess I was having what people in the old days used to refer to as a "nervous breakdown."

Now I'm not sure what a "nervous breakdown" is, so I just like to call that the day I had my "break." It wasn't a break from reality; rather, it was just the day my brain and body said, "No more." My poor husband had so much on his mind that week that he really didn't understand what was going on. He kept thinking I was just going to get up and go back to work. I'd inform him that I wasn't going back, and he'd keep asking me why not. He just didn't understand at the time.

Finally, about four weeks later, I went up to the school and turned in my resignation from the school district. At the same time, I applied for state disability retirement. This is where I applied to be eligible to claim disability from the state retirement system that I had paid into for the last 14 years. Luckily, it came through about six weeks later.

During those four weeks before I resigned, I had another stint as an inpatient in a psychiatric facility for my depression. It was horrible. That was my 5th time as an inpatient in about two and a half years. But I was still just popping my pills and acting as if my mental illness were a head cold or something I didn't need to address, even though it had cost me my job, my doctorate, and just about everything else.

Fast forward about three years… There had been more depression, a couple of bouts of mania accompanied with wild shopping sprees and money spending, and finally, another inpatient hospitalization for depression. This time I missed my daughter's dance recital AND my son's baseball tournament all in the same week. In return, I got to sit in group sessions and tell people how I felt. I got to eat institution food. I got to wake up at six in the morning and share a room with someone I didn't know. (She turned out to be very nice.) I got to miss my favorite television shows and give up access to my cell phone and computer. I also had to give up access to my family and friends—all so a doctor I didn't know could play with my meds, and nurses I didn't know could poke and prod me. One nurse even had the nerve to tell me that I took so much medication that she could hear me rattle every time I walked down the hall (I filed a complaint against her, although I doubt that anything came of it.)

Ouch! Something changed during that hospitalization. It finally dawned on me that I didn't want to do that anymore. I didn't want to go back there. I didn't want to be hospitalized. I didn't want to get to the point anymore that I required hospitalization to get my meds straightened out. If my medicines were starting to slip, why couldn't I or someone close to me recognize that at home? Why did it have to get to this point before I made a change?

And then it dawned on me.

I made a decision.

I grew up in the Deep South where a lot of people I knew were Southern Baptists. I was raised Episcopalian, but I always found it interesting that for Southern Baptists, they were required to "make a conscious decision" for Jesus and walk down the aisle to be "saved." I kind of had an epiphany like that, but it wasn't about anything religious.

Before I came home from the hospital that last time in June of 2009, I made a conscious decision that I was NOT going back to the hospital anymore—not unless I had some kind of physical illness that required immediate and acute medical attention. I decided then and there that my mental health was going to be the most important thing in my life—more important than my kids, my friends, more important than anything. It would be my first priority. I would do whatever it took to be sure that I stayed mentally healthy. I would talk about it. I would advocate for myself. I would surround myself with people who would advocate for me and act in my best interest and tell me if they saw the first sign of me acting weird, inappropriate, or just plain "off." I was going to do all that I could to stay healthy.

Nobody could do this but me.

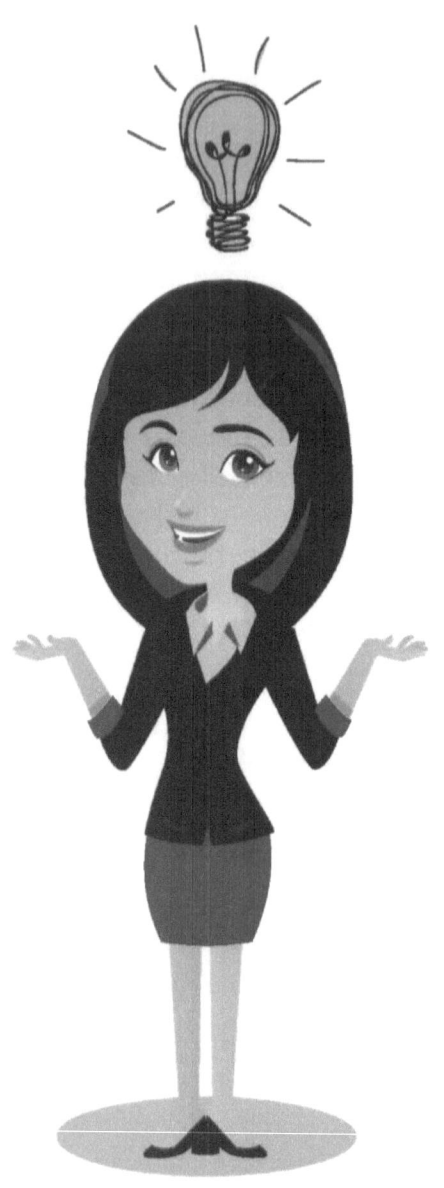

CHAPTER 3

Making Peace with the "Beast"

After having had my epiphany, I realized that in order to get better and *stay* better, I'd have to not only acknowledge that I was mentally ill, but I'd have to completely accept that my illness was a part of my everyday life, rather than an occasional distraction. Furthermore, this illness was going to be with me for the rest of my years. I couldn't dress it up with a few pills each day and hide it in the corner like I'd been trying to do for the past 15 years or so. (Ironically, my playing "dress up" with it had caused it to come out more than it had hidden it, so obviously that game hadn't been working!)

Nope. This time I was going to have to accept that I, Laura Gray, had a mental illness that lived in my brain and affected my personality and actions. I could medicate it, and I could take steps to minimize it, but I would never be able to make it completely disappear.

And you know what? Once I finally wrapped my head around that idea, another idea came to me: I wasn't my mental illness. I wasn't "bipolar." You know how someone might say, "Oh yeah, that's Laura over there. She's bipolar." It occurred to me that this statement just wasn't true. I wasn't bipolar and everything that bipolar disorder embodied. Nor was I OCD and everything that obsessive-compulsive disorder embodied. I wasn't even ADD and everything that adult attention deficit disorder embodied. I wasn't my illness at all—or even the sum total of all of my diagnoses. I was just Laura who had these illnesses, just like Laura might have a cold or Laura might have allergies or hay fever. I wasn't my disease. I was a person who just happened to have an illness or two, and a very treatable illness at that!

That was probably THE most freeing moment that I can ever remember in my life. Now I'm very careful to correct people close to me who say things like, "Yeah, he's schizophrenic" or "She's bipolar." I tell them that you certainly wouldn't walk around saying, "Oh, look at Sally. She's cancer," so why say that someone is the embodiment of their mental illness? No, that person is just a person who happens to have a mental illness—he's not the sum total of his illness.

Once I learned to separate myself from my illness, it was much, much easier for me to accept that I had an illness. And then, after accepting that I had an illness, I was able to learn about it with much more objectivity. It wasn't all doom and gloom and a horrible prognosis anymore. I learned that my disease is quite manageable and quite treatable. I also learned that it was not necessary for me to go inpatient when I needed a medication tweak or adjustment. In fact, it wasn't even necessary for me to get to the point where I was in crisis anymore. With help, I could actually moderate my own moods and feelings so that I never had to have a crisis episode or "breakdown" ever again! (Wow!)

And after I accepted my illness and could admit to myself that I had a treatable and manageable mental health diagnosis, I discovered that I didn't mind so much admitting any of that to other people. Of course, I wasn't comfortable enough at that point to shout it from the rooftops, but I didn't deny it to anybody either, as I had for the last 15+ years. It gradually became no big deal. Some people had diabetes. Others had high blood pressure or acne. I had a mental illness. No biggie.

At the point that I "came out of the closet" and started talking about it to a few people here and there, another interesting thing happened. Because it wasn't such a big deal to me, I discovered that it wasn't such a big deal to other people either. Some people were really surprised to find this out about me. Others had already figured it out even though I had worked very, very hard to hide it. They had put two and two together a long time ago. Either way, hardly anyone seemed to care, and of the very few who did, I decided I didn't want those people in my life anyway. I haven't missed them since, but I have found out that many of my friends eventually cut these same people out of their lives for a variety of reasons, so obviously they weren't stellar friends anyway.

Accepting my illness was really easy compared to making peace with myself. That part took much longer to do.

I have come to believe that the act of making peace with oneself, no matter what one is making peace over, is a process. It's not something that happens overnight or even quickly. For me, accepting my illness came quickly; it just swept over me, and the things that happened afterward rolled in like waves rolling onto the shore. Making peace with yourself doesn't work like that—at least it never has worked that way for me.

I think the reason for this is because I'm a perfectionist and hold myself to such a high standard. I've been told more than once (and my husband would most certainly tell you) that I hold others to high standards, but I hold myself to impossibly high standards. There is a great deal of truth in this statement. So, when it came to making peace with myself over having a mental illness, it was a very difficult process for me... not because I felt that I should have been perfect and illness-free, but because I felt that I had failed by not accepting my illness much earlier in my life and that I felt that I had failed by allowing my illness to control my life for as long as it had. In other words, had I only done this ten or twelve years sooner, I could have achieved so much more and have had such a happier life leading up to the time when I did accept my illness.

Now… you and I both know that this is completely irrational thinking. And trust me—I now know that it took the sum total of everything happening exactly the way that it did in my life (and at the time that it did) for me to get to where I am right now, which is a pretty damned happy and successful place. However, at the time I didn't know this, and I actually thought that I was a failure for not having come to this realization soon enough despite the fact that it took everything happening exactly the way it did to get me to the point where I *could* accept my illness and make peace with myself. (Was I crazy or what back then???)

So…in addition to having bipolar illness, OCD, and ADD, evidently I was suffering from an unrelenting case of perfectionism, which I still have to keep in check from time to time, by the way. It took quite a bit of therapy and a good talking down from both my husband and a couple of good friends to get me to the point where I could say to myself, "Hey! You know what? It's really okay that you're just now accepting all of this. And it's okay that it took everything it took to get you to this point. You're alive, you've got a great husband and three wonderful kids, and your life may not be perfect, but under the circumstances, it's pretty damned good. So chill, and be grateful."

And at that point, I learned about gratitude. I started counting my blessings rather than wishing for the unobtainable. Acceptance, peace with myself, and gratitude had become my daily practices. And that's when I sat down and formulated the steps that would be my path to recovery.

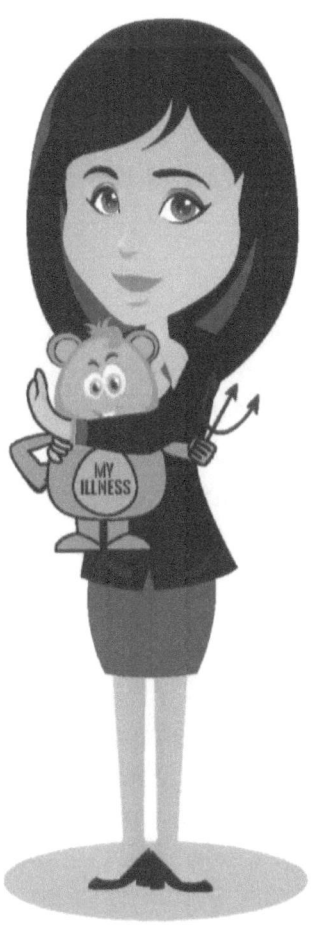

CHAPTER 4

Mental Health Issues and Genetics: The Luck of the Draw

I never asked to have a mental illness. Chances are, you probably didn't either. Even if you've just been dealing with depression or anxiety, they still fall under the umbrella term of "mental illnesses," so we'll collectively call them that. Don't worry... it's not meant as a derogatory term; this is only to separate these illnesses (and they ARE truly illnesses) from non brain-based illness such as diabetes, kidney stones, heart disease, high blood pressure, and the like.

So, back to mental illness. You didn't ask for it. I didn't ask for it. Our friends and families certainly didn't ask for us to have it. Where did this come from? For starters, you can probably blame a family member. The research out there shows that there is a strong genetic component when it comes to illnesses such as depression, anxiety, bipolar disorder, schizoaffective disorder, schizophrenia, obsessive-compulsive disorder (which falls on the anxiety spectrum, but more about that later), and the like.

My father was a raging alcoholic, and from the time I was nine or ten until he died when I was twenty-seven, he self-medicated his bipolar disorder with alcohol. Although he was never formally diagnosed, from what I know from his family members, his personality dating back to the time he was a teenager was always either way "on" or way "off." When he was "on," he spent money like crazy and drank to excess, and when he was "off," he drank even more and displayed inappropriate anger—clearly signs of typical bipolar mood swings. It wasn't much of a stretch, then, for me to realize that genetics was, indeed, at play when I was diagnosed with bipolar disorder at the age of twenty-one.

It was a year later that I discovered, quite by accident, that my mother had depression. On my twenty-second birthday, she decided to quit smoking. While she and I were both very grateful that she chose to do this, she soon realized that she had been using nicotine for many years to mask her symptoms of clinical depression. That made two people in the family.

Less than a year after my mother found that she had depression and began treatment for it, my dad's mother asked me a very strange question one day as I was visiting her in rural north Louisiana. Keep in mind that I didn't see her very often—maybe once a year—but I had taken a trip out there overnight one weekend, mainly to see my dad's sister, whom I adored, and I had stopped by my granny's house to eat dinner and visit that evening. She and I were sitting in the kitchen having a cup of coffee, and she asked me out of the blue, "Laura, do you ever just feel really down and depressed? I do sometimes."

I was floored. See, my granny and I had never been really close. We just didn't talk about things like that. She didn't know my mental health history or anything about my recent diagnosis. We didn't talk about my dad's alcoholism. We didn't talk about my parents' divorce. In short, we just didn't talk about anything of substance. Everything with her was superficial. Until she asked me that question. I looked at her and said, "Yes, yes I do. I feel that way a lot. In fact, I take medicine for it." She asked if the medicine made me feel better, and I told her it did. She didn't say another word about it, and the subject never came up again. I saw her maybe once more after that, and she died two or three years later. I'll never know what prompted to ask me that, why she felt depressed, or what the source of that depression was, but I'm inclined to believe that maybe she suffered from depression, too. And so there were three.

Of course, over the years, I've learned that depression, anxiety, and bipolar disorder (even though my diagnosis has been changed to schizoaffective disorder in the last three years) are all over my family. My husband and one of my children suffer from anxiety. One deals with social anxiety, and the other deals with generalized anxiety. My husband also deals with depression, as do two of my children. Another of my children suffers from bipolar disorder, and two of the kids were diagnosed with ADHD at a young age. I myself, am the poster child for Adult ADD. So, you see, we're just full of diagnoses at our house.

You're probably thinking by now, "Gee, Laura... you must really have your hands full!" Well... truthfully, we're pretty much a normal family. The only difference is that we do what I described in the previous chapter. We take care of ourselves. We advocate for ourselves and one another. We take our medicine, just as someone with diabetes would take his insulin or just as a person with high blood pressure would take her medicine. We make sure we get enough sleep, eat at the proper times, control stress as much as possible, etc. We do what it takes to stay healthy, heredity be damned.

The other thing that may be crossing your mind is, "If you knew that there was a genetic component, why did you have three children?" That's a legitimate question. I did know there was a genetic component. The first answer to that question is that I wanted to be a mother, and I wanted to have children. I also wanted more than one child because I was an only child, and that wasn't much fun. The second answer, and the "real" answer, is that I know I'm a survivor, and I knew that if any of my children ended up with a mental illness, I could deal with it and teach them how to be survivors, too. End of story. So yes, I purposely had kids, and I have absolutely no regrets.

Now… about heredity. As with many other diseases, the up side to being diagnosed with a mental illness is that you can most likely trace its origins in your family tree somewhere. The down side is also that you can trace its origins in your family tree somewhere, and that if you have biological children, there's a likelihood that at least one of them has a good chance of presenting with the same illness that you do. But hey—that's true of many, many diseases, and the vast majority of mental illnesses are very treatable nowadays, and if you practice good self-care and self-advocacy, your prognosis is good.

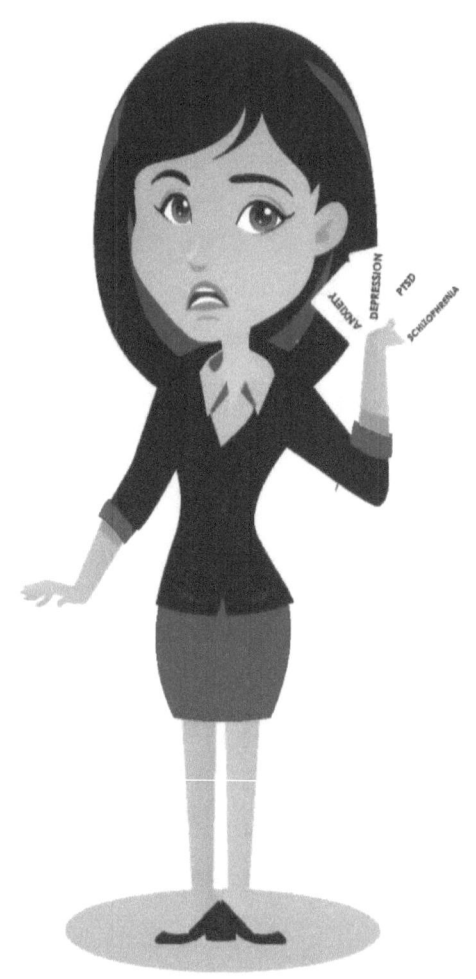

CHAPTER 5

What's Happening in My Brain???

If I haven't said this plainly as of yet, let me say this very, very plainly right now: Depression, Anxiety, Obsessive-Compulsive Disorder, Bipolar Disorder, Schizoaffective Disorder, Shizophrenia, PTSD... all these things... They're not something you can just "pull yourself up by the bootstraps" and get over. You just can't magically wish yourself to feel better, and POOF! You feel better. You can't try harder, and they're gone. They're BRAIN DISEASES. Yes, you heard me correctly. Brain diseases. Brain illnesses. In other words, physical illnesses that people like to call "mental illnesses" because they affect your psyche. But something is PHYSICALLY wrong with your brain. Read my lips: YOUR BRAIN IS NOT WORKING CORRECTLY, AND THIS IS WHY YOU HAVE THIS ILLNESS.

There is nothing—-nothing whatsoever—that you or anyone else has done to cause this. Yes, there are triggers for depression and anxiety, and especially for PTSD. There are also times in our lives when we are more susceptible to these illnesses showing up. The teenage and young adult years, for example, are the prime time for many, if not most, of these illnesses to manifest. And if they don't show up then, for women, pre-menopause is another time that it can happen.

So…you've got a mental/brain/physical illness. What, exactly, is happening in your brain to cause this? I wanted to know the same thing, too, so I contacted someone on my health care team, my wonderful psychiatrist, Dr. Alonso. Dr. Alonso is from Mexico City, and he's not only a great psychiatrist, but he also specializes in neuropsychiatry, which means that he is intimately familiar with all of the inner workings of the brain as it relates to mental illness, AND he can explain these things so that the average layperson (like me) can understand it.

There are three main neurotransmitters, or brain chemicals, that are involved in mental illnesses. They are norepinephrine, serotonin, and dopamine. We'll talk about norepinephrine first.

Norepinephrine, which in addition to being a neurotransmitter, is also a hormone, and it is associated with a number of things. The thing that most people associate it with is giving us a burst of energy in very stressful situations. In other words, it's commonly associated with the "fight or flight" syndrome. However, when someone suffers from depression, he or she often doesn't have enough norepinephrine. This is what causes the slow-moving, slow response, flattened affect (or lack of expressiveness), and seemingly "down" mood that we see in people who are depressed. This happens because the depressed person doesn't have enough of a "pick-me-up" chemical in his or her body.

While it is not really known what causes a shortage of norepinephrine in most depressed people, one thing that is known is that people who have dealt with prolonged extreme stress (such as combat or the prolonged critical illness of a loved one, for example) are more prone to chronic depression because it is believed that they have depleted their own norepinephrine levels in the brain.

Regardless of the cause of the shortage of norepinephrine, the treatment for depression due to low norepinephrine is most often an antidepressant that increases norepinephrine levels in the brain. With this increase in norepinephrine, the depressed person will show signs of relief and recovery. Of course, talk therapy as an adjunct treatment is also advisable.

A second brain chemical dealing with depression and other mood disorders is serotonin, also known as "the happy chemical," as it has been believed for many years to contribute to happiness and well-being. Serotonin got worldwide attention back in 1986 when the first SSRI, or Selective Serotonin Reuptake Inhibitor, better known as Prozac, hit the pharmaceutical market. Prozac was touted as the latest, greatest thing to hit pharmacy shelves, and it literally revolutionized psychiatry and the treatment of depression. It has been used not only to treat depression, but also obsessive-compulsive disorder, bulimia, alcohol dependency, obesity, post-traumatic stress disorder, and a host of other illnesses and disorders, and it has been deemed relatively safe for use in pregnancy and breastfeeding (Pregnancy Category B). As of 2016, there were over 23 million Prozac users in the United States alone!

Needless to say, after the introduction of Prozac, SSRIs became the "gold standard" for the treatment of these illnesses and many others. They work by simply blocking the reuptake, or reabsorption, of serotonin in the brain. It is believed that when one suffers from any of the above-mentioned illnesses, it is because their serotonin doesn't quite get where it's supposed to go by transmitting signals from one nerve cell to the other. Ideally, it transmits these signals by moving across a "synapse" to get to the next nerve cell. In a person with depression (or OCD or PTSD, let's say), before the serotonin can cross the synapse, it is reabsorbed, so it never does transmit the intended signal to the next nerve cell. SSRIs work by giving serotonin the extra "push" that it needs to send its signals without being reabsorbed, thus causing a shortage of it in the brain. Make sense?

Now we'll move onto the third neurotransmitter, called dopamine. Dopamine is the brain chemical commonly associated with pleasure, although it controls many other things, as well. Dopamine deficiency can lead to serious depression, schizophrenia, schizoaffective disorder, hallucinations, psychosis, and even Parkinson's Disease. Dopamine works in the brain in much the same way that serotonin does; it sends signals to nerve cells across synapses. Therefore, dopamine reuptake inhibitors such as bupropion (Wellbutrin is its trade name) work to relieve depression caused by a dopamine shortage in the brain. Because so many illnesses with psychotic features stem from not having enough dopamine, the vast majority of antipsychotic medications work on dopamine receptors in one way or another, although the "atypical" antipsychotics are newer and are less likely to cause some of the nastier side effects rendered by the older, or "typical" antipsychotics.

Now that we've taken a look at the three main neurotransmitters, or brain chemicals, that are associated with mental illness, as well as what goes on in the brain with these chemicals when we become ill, it is important to remember that we cannot presume to diagnose ourselves if and when we do begin to suffer from one or more of these illnesses. While it's great to have some knowledge about what is going on within our bodies and about the names of the chemicals responsible, it is always best to leave the diagnosis of our illness(es) and the treatment to a medically trained, board certified psychiatrist or psychiatric nurse practitioner who works under the watchful eye of a psychiatrist.

These are the people who have been trained and who have put their life's work into diagnosing and treating these illnesses. These are the people who stay up-to-date on all of the latest psychotropic medicines on the market and who know which ones treat which symptoms and act on which specific neurotransmitters. And while I'm not suggesting at all that you don't do research about your illness or the meds prescribed to you or even about your doctor's background and field of expertise, I am suggesting that you leave the real nitty-gritty scientific stuff to him or her.

That being said, though, you can, and should, make it your business to know a bit about your brain and about the chemicals (or lack of chemicals, as it were) that are probably responsible for your illness. Remember: mental illness isn't something you can just snap out of or get up out of bed and suddenly "do better" with. It's a bona fide illness with physical origins. And the physical origins are the ones we just talked about in this chapter (and likely many others in addition to these). So... the next time one of your well-meaning "friends" sees that you're having a bad day and tells you to "deal with it" or that you should just "do better," be sure to tell this "friend" about the neurotransmitter shortage in your brain. Read a bit more online, and go into great detail. That ought to shut him up! ;-)

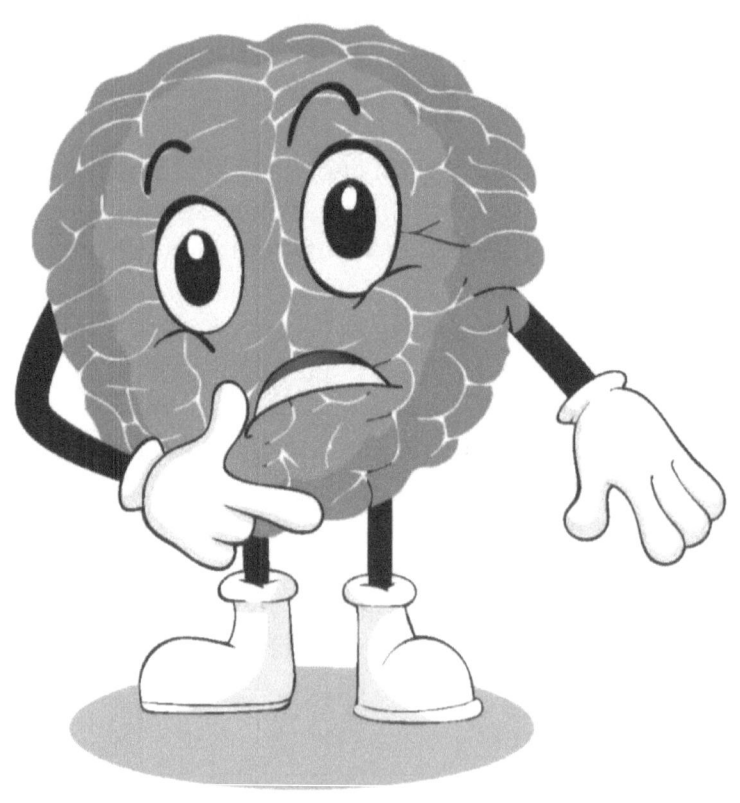

CHAPTER 6

Now… About Those Five Simple Steps…

Like I said earlier, it occurred to me after that last hospitalization that I did NOT want to ever go back to that again. I decided then and there to do whatever it took to prevent finding myself in that state of mind again. At the time, I had no idea that there were five specific steps I needed to take to prevent it—heck, I didn't know how many steps there were or what those steps would look like, but I knew I needed to make some major changes in my life and do SOMETHING to keep it happening again. Obviously, what I had been doing for the last several years hadn't been working so well.

One thing I hadn't done at all was to accept that I had a mental illness. Oh, I knew that I had been diagnosed with bipolar disorder when I was 21, and I knew I'd had problems with depression since I was about 14 and all that, but I had pretty much brushed it aside all these years. I very blissfully operated under the assumption that as long as I took my medicine every day and occasionally popped in to see a therapist (who changed often—and I mean *really* often), I could function just fine—just like everyone else, right? (Wrong.)

Nope. I had to truly acknowledge that this illness was a part of me, and not only wasn't it going to go away, but it couldn't be swept under the rug either. It really did affect every part of my life, and during the times when it had reared its ugly head and had required me to undergo hospitalization, it had disrupted not only my life, but the lives of my entire family and close friends as well. And that wasn't cool.

So... that was the first thing I had to do. Then it occurred to me that acknowledging my illness meant maybe, just maybe, that I'd have to talk about it. I had never done that before. I hadn't even really talked about it to anybody, not even my husband. It's like it had been this deep, dark secret that I'd been hiding for the past twenty or so years. This was really ironic because all this time, I had acted so indignant about people putting labels on people who were mentally ill and stigmatizing them, and as it turns out, I had been doing the very same thing by hiding my illness and being ashamed of it. This was a tough lesson for me, and it didn't feel good to figure this out.

Once I had done that, the first thing I had to do was to come to the realization that I was ultimately in charge of the medicines I took, and it was up to me to put together a health care team whom I liked and trusted and with whom I was comfortable working. This realization hit me a couple of weeks after I was released from the hospital. I had a follow-up appointment with my psychiatrist at the time, and while I was sitting across from her in her office, a thought occurred to me. "I don't really like her," I realized. "She seems to be stuck on prescribing a lot of old medicines and doesn't seem to be really up on the new stuff that's out there. Furthermore, she doesn't seem to be concerned about side effects."

I'll admit that I've always had a "thing" about my weight, and over the last couple of years at that time, I had put on a good seventy pounds, which I think was largely due to the medicines I was taking. When I had tried to bring this up to my doctor, she had just shrugged it off, stating that if I wanted to feel better, this was something I would have to put up with. So when I got out of the hospital on new and different medications, I began to research the side effects and see which ones promoted weight gain and which ones didn't, and it occurred to me that maybe I had a choice in which medicines I took. Maybe it was possible to take meds for my particular symptoms that did *not* cause weight gain. Unfortunately, she wouldn't hear of it. I decided then and there that it was time for a change of psychiatrists.

Fortunately, I really liked my therapist. She and I got along very well even though she was a no-nonsense kind of lady. I never did like the touchy-feely types who always wanted to ask me, "How do you feel about that?" Yuck. I told my therapist at the time this, and she said that if she ever had to ask me how I felt about something, she wasn't doing her job right. Sold! I've operated under that mantra ever since, and no matter where I've lived since, I've gotten along a-okay with my therapists.

So, it took a bit of time and some work, but I finally put together the perfect psychiatrist, therapist, and family practice doctor (whom I had seen for years and years) for me. I made sure that each knew about the others, and even though it wasn't the normal practice for doctors and therapists to communicate, I made sure that each of them had the others' contact information should they need to be in touch with one another. In addition, I always kept them abreast of my appointments with the other two. I figured that was my responsibility as the patient.

The second thing I needed to do was to find a good support system. (I'm not talking about a support group.) What I mean is a group of several people with whom I was very close who would help me, by pointing out if I seemed to be having several bad days in a row or seemed kind of "off," to discern whether or not I maybe needed a med tweak or change or an appointment RIGHT NOW with my psychiatrist or therapist.

I've never been the type to have lots of close friends, but this didn't prove to be as difficult as I thought it would.

The third thing I decided to do was to start taking better care of myself. This is something I'd neglected for quite a long time—really, since I was in college back in the late 80's and early 90's. It occurred to me that I would feel much better if I slept well each night, regulated my eating (I was bad to skip a meal or two and then eat a HUGE meal to make up for it), exercised a bit, and systematically cut stressful situations and people out of my life.

This was a bit more difficult for me. At least the part about cutting out stressful people and situations was. For one thing, having grown up in an alcoholic household, all I really knew and understood was stress and chaos. So, in the absence of any stress and chaos, I had been one to manufacture stressful and chaotic situations. (This is NOT a good thing to do, by the way, as it affects everyone around you!) However, I was eventually able to do this, and life has been much better since.

Fourth, I knew I had to obtain some balance in my life. Again, I was someone who had voluntarily taken seven or eight classes at a time during my undergraduate years, was an officer in several clubs and a member of at least as many more, and worked nearly full-time. (Not good either. Are you seeing a pattern here?) When I was working as an adult, I was essentially doing the same thing, too. And then, when I had to stop working altogether, I literally went from doing way, way too much to doing absolutely nothing. There had to be something in-between.

The fifth thing on my list came later on, maybe several years later. Once I had gotten myself stable, healthy, and in a good place, I knew that I had to advocate not only for myself but also for others who weren't as strong as I was. I began to research volunteer groups who catered to the mentally ill, and I joined a couple of Facebook support groups for those who had mental health issues. There I was able to assist people who needed help but who weren't strong enough to speak with their own voices just yet. In the meantime, I made sure that when I needed to advocate for myself, that I could and did. It's a very satisfying and powerful feeling to be able to do that, and each time I do speak up for myself or someone who can't, I'm reminded of the time when I couldn't, and it humbles me.

Was completing these five steps easy? No, not necessarily. But they were simple, not complicated at all. I didn't do anything convoluted, drawn-out, or impossible. And I wouldn't ask anybody else to do something convoluted, drawn-out, or impossible either. These steps are entirely doable. It may take you several months to accomplish getting them done, or it may take you a few years, like it did me, but they are certainly doable.

In the next five chapters, I'll go into detail about each step and will discuss some of the common pitfalls and complications that are possible with each, so you can go all in…armed and ready!

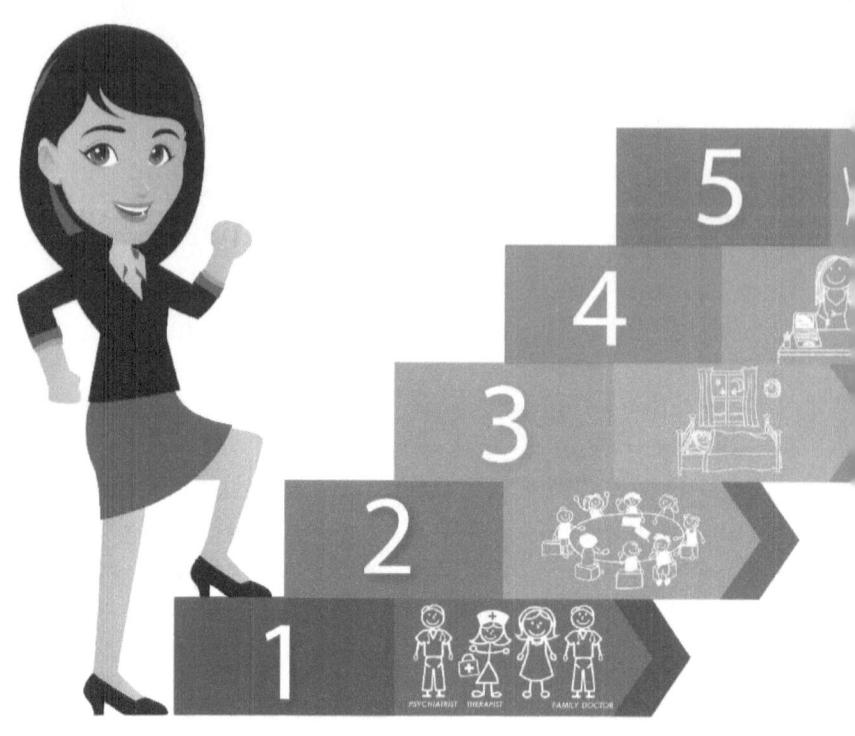

CHAPTER 7

Step 1: Putting Together a Winning Mental Health Team

For the majority of people, when they get sick enough to go to the doctor, they call and make an appointment, take the next appointment that's available according to what the person on the other end of the phone line tells them, and they show up at the appointed time for their appointment. They may have to wait only 15 or 20 minutes to see the doctor, or they may have to wait upwards of two or more hours to get to the back to be seen. Regardless, when they do get to see the doctor, they tell him or her what's wrong, the doctor looks them over and maybe asks a few questions, sometimes orders a blood test or an x-ray (or maybe more), and generally writes at least one prescription.

Only rarely does the patient ask questions about the prescription other than to verify how often to take said medicine throughout the day and for how many days. In fact, much of the time, when questioned about exactly which medicine he or she was given by the doctor, the sick person can't even tell the person doing the asking any of the details. The answer usually goes something like this: "Oh, I don't remember. It was some antibiotic." Or "It's a green pill. I can't remember what it's called." And, as if like there's nothing in the world wrong with that, we nod, smile, and accept these answers as if they're perfectly okay.

But have you ever stopped to think that these answers maybe aren't okay? That perhaps we have not only the right— but also the responsibility—to know what we're taking? Yes. We do. We also have the responsibility to know what the side effects of the drug are, who manufactures it, which drugs AND foods and drinks it might interfere with, and most important of all: WHY we were prescribed the drug in the first place and WHAT it's supposed to do to our bodies.

But wait, you say! Isn't the doctor supposed to tell us all that? Well yes… perhaps. Maybe. But as smart consumers, it's our responsibility to make it our business to find out about these things in the case that 1. The doctor is busy/forgetful/confused/new/not well-versed on that drug and doesn't tell us, and 2. It's our bodies the drug is going into, not the doctor's, so it's our responsibility to know these things.

That, my friends, is called being a smart consumer!

So... why did I lead this chapter with a lecture on being a smart consumer?

Well... in order to take Step 1 and put together a winning health care team—YOUR winning health care team (because your winning health care team may be vastly different than mine or someone else's), you must first dedicate yourself to being a smart consumer. Why, you ask? That's easy. Because YOU are the number one person on your winning health care team! Yes, you read that correctly. You are a part of your health care team. You get to be a part of the decisions that are made about your health care. Not only do you have a right to be a part of this decision-making team, but you have an OBLIGATION to be a part of it.

Gone are the days where people will be making these decisions in your absence. Gone are the days where your children, your parents, or your spouse will be deciding, along with your doctor, that it's time for you to have another inpatient visit because your meds are off-kilter again. Those days are over. I am hereby giving you the power to be an integral part of your own health care team and to help make your own decisions regarding your mental health.

By your stepping up to the plate and being the #1 person on your team, you have committed to you and your health care team that nobody is letting you get into crisis mode again. You may need the occasional medicinal tweak, and you may have a bad day here and there, but you're committing to putting your mental health first—making it your number one priority—and doing all that you (and your team) can to see that you don't slip into crisis mode again! Wow! Doesn't that feel great? Doesn't it?!?

Now... Let's talk about how we can put this Dream Team together.

First, you'll need a psychiatrist or a nurse practitioner who is overseen by a psychiatrist. Here are the things that I, personally, look for in a psychiatrist or NP.

1. I don't want someone who's on the verge of retirement. I'd like the person I see to be around for awhile.

2. I don't mind working with a nurse practitioner either. In fact, there are some very, very good ones out there. And, in this day and age of a major shortage of psychiatrists, this may be the path you go down whether you intend to or not!

3. I'm not picky about whether my person is male or female. If you have a preference, don't settle. Be true to yourself.

4. I am insistent—absolutely insistent—that my health care provider know, unequivocally, that I *am* going to have a voice in my care, ask questions, and offer input. While I don't presume to know medicine, I am a smart girl, and I do keep up with my research on psychotropic meds. I am a well-informed consumer. If you're the same way, and your doctor doesn't like or allow that, GO ELSEWHERE.

5. There are certain kinds of meds that I will not take. For example, I won't take antipsychotics (or any other drugs) that make me gain weight. Will.Not.Do.It. It's a non-starter. I'm aware that there are a few out there that don't cause weight gain, I know what the side-effects and risks are, and I've done my homework on them. My doctor and I have come to an

agreement on these. Again, if your doctor tells you that you HAVE to take a certain medicine that you feel is a non-starter for you, GO ELSEWHERE. There are hundreds of psychotropic drugs on the market, and there is ALWAYS an option!

And remember, it's okay to make a short appointment with a psychiatrist or a nurse practitioner just to interview him and see what he's like. You may need to pay for that visit out of pocket, but it is so worth it in the end to find someone with whom you really "click." Don't be nervous. Tell him what you're looking for in a doctor. Tell him you want to be a partner in your health care. Tell him you're committed to staying out of crisis and that your mental health is the most important thing in your life. I promise he'll be impressed-- because the majority of his patients are NOT like that!

Now that you've found a good psychiatrist or NP who is supervised by a psychiatrist, the next step is to find a good therapist.

Here's what I look for in a therapist:

Now remember…These are MY preferences. Just mine. They don't have to be yours or anybody else's. This is just an illustration of how you do have the right to be a bit choosy when it comes to your health care team. In the past ten years, when I have met with a therapist to interview him or her (and it makes no difference to me whether that therapist is male or female, although it may to you), I tell him:

1. I am not a "hugger." In other words, please don't get touchy-feely with me. It makes me uncomfortable.

2. Please don't ask me to keep a journal or suggest that I meditate. I know how to relax, and I'm quite good at it. I'm

also good at expressing my feelings and at identifying my feelings. I positively loathe journaling, as I do a great deal of writing for a living, so I don't want to spend my non-working hours writing.

3. Don't ask me, "How do you feel about _____?" I speak my mind, so if, after talking with me for 10 or 15 minutes, you aren't sure how I feel about something, then you're not doing your job!

I also prefer to see a therapist who doesn't run constantly behind with his or her patients. One of my pet peeves is feeling as if somebody is wasting my time, so if I have to sit and wait for over 30 minutes to see my therapist—especially on a day when I'm not feeling so great—I'm going to feel angry and resentful about that, and I will probably take it out on you, the therapist. Punctuality is a big plus in my book, and I can overlook other issues so long as my therapist is relatively punctual.

All that aside, I do prefer a therapist who gets straight to the point with me. If I'm sitting there spewing utter bullshit, I want my therapist to call me on it and tell me, "Laura, that's bullshit, and you know it!" In other words, keep me accountable, and don't let me get away with anything! I can manipulate others as well as anyone else can. I learned how to do it at an early age (after all, I grew up with an alcoholic father), and I figure if my therapist doesn't recognize that and stop me, I'm not getting my money's worth. I want to be held accountable, I want to be challenged, and I want to grow. Basically, I want to leave each session a little bit better of a person than when I walked in. Otherwise, like I said, I'm not getting my money's worth.

So… we've got a great psychiatrist/NP and a therapist who ticks all the boxes. What next?

Now we need a regular, general practice or family doctor (or internist) who can take care of our everyday sicknesses.

But why, you may ask, should this person be a part of THAT health care team?

Here's the short answer: It's all about communication. Each of these three people should not only know your history and what's going on with you, but they should be able to communicate with one another should a crisis arise, as well. In addition, each of them should know exactly which medicines you're taking for what.

Here's an illustration. My family doctor prescribes my thyroid medicine and my estrogen (I'm several years post-hysterectomy, so I take hormone replacement. No judgment, please. It's what's best for me.) My psychiatrist doesn't prescribe these meds, nor is it his job. On the other hand, my psychiatrist prescribes my anti-depressant, my anti-psychotic, my mood stabilizer, etc. My family doctor knows something about these drugs and how they work, but my psychiatrist is far more qualified to monitor these medicines than she is. However, they both need to know about everything I take in case one of them prescribes something for me that could interfere with a medicine that the other one prescribes. Make sense?

Besides, I look at it this way: I want as many people in my corner as possible, and if that means three competent professionals who are concerned about my mental health and well-being and who are looking out for my welfare, then so be it. Also, with three people watching over me, one of them is bound to see a glitch in the system (the "system" being me) before I do, and the quicker someone sees it and identifies said glitch, the quicker we can go about fixing it before it develops into a full-blown crisis!

There have been two times that I can recall in which my family doctor has noticed that something was "off kilter" with me well before I was due to see my psychiatrist. In fact, the last time it happened, I had just come from a meeting with my therapist the day before, and I, myself, thought that everything was okay. I had been feeling a bit tired and run-down lately and couldn't explain why. I was sleeping an hour or so more at night than normal, and while I didn't feel depressed, per se, I wasn't my usual happy, chipper self. After I explained this to my family practice doctor and she had examined me, she asked me a few more questions. Because she was well aware of my psychiatric history and knew which antidepressant I was currently taking—as well as which I had previously been on over the last several years—she started asking me questions such as when I had last upped my dosage, how long I had been on that particular medicine, and so on. To make a long story short, I was beginning to show early signs of depression, and it was, indeed, time to see my psychiatrist for a medication tweak.

She was able to call my psychiatrist from her office—right then—and let his office secretary know that I needed to see him sooner rather than later. (These kinds of calls carry much more clout when they come from other doctors than when you, the patient, call and say the same thing. It shouldn't be that way, but it is.) Luckily, I was able to get in to see my psychiatrist the very next day to get that small dosage change and a new prescription for the larger dose, so I avoided several weeks of feeling "off," as well as an impending crisis, by having my family doctor on my health care team. Laura's Health Care Team-1, Mental Health Crisis-0.

Let me just say here that not everybody puts together a winning health care team on the first try. It often takes time and effort to find the well-oiled machine of a team that works for you. Life tends to get in the way, too. We change jobs and consequently have to change insurance plans. Sometimes we move to a new state or even to a new country. Doctors and therapists retire or stop accepting our insurance. Things happen. But trust me when I say that there IS more than one psychiatrist/nurse practitioner, therapist, and family doctor/general practitioner/internist out there for you!

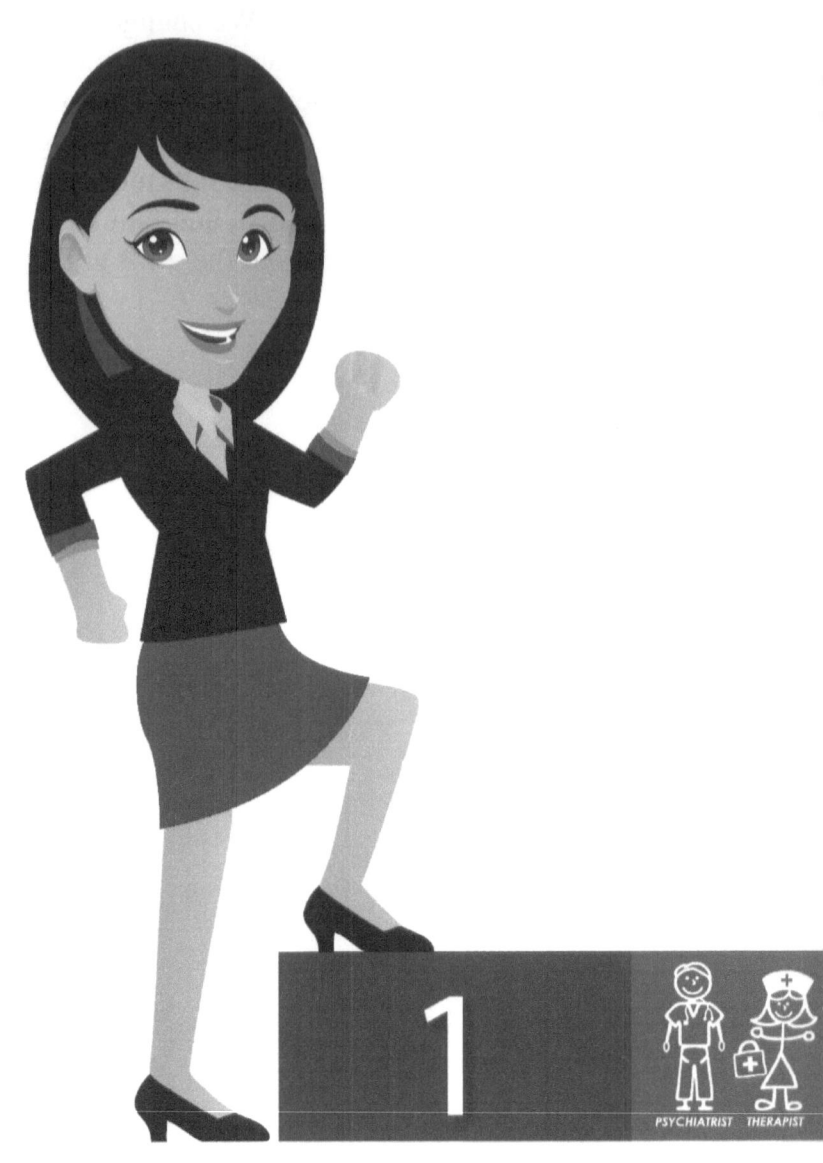

CHAPTER 8

Step 2: Finding Your Support System—And Using It!

It's not enough to have a great mental health team on your side. No... you also need your own support system to win at the mental health game. I'm not necessarily talking about a support group, per se, although if you feel that you would benefit from attending a support group for depression, anxiety, bipolar disorder, or general mental health issues, they can certainly be helpful and supportive. Keep in mind, though, that everyone in these groups has also been diagnosed with either the same thing you have or something similar, and each of these people has his or her own mental health issues to deal with, so they can only be as supportive as their own illnesses allow them to be.

When I say that you need a support system, I'm talking about a core group of five to seven people with whom you are pretty close and whom you see and/or communicate with on a regular basis. In other words, people who know you well and who can identify when you're just not "yourself." People who would notice when you're having a hard time. And most important of all, people who would not hesitate to tell you that you're just not yourself and that you seem to be having a rough go of it.

Now don't panic. I'm not suggesting AT ALL that you go out and round up a group of people who would readily commit you to an inpatient psychiatric facility at the slightest hint that you were having an "off" day. Actually, I'm suggesting just the opposite. The purpose of your support system is to keep you OUT of the hospital! How, you ask? By noticing when you are first showing signs of being a bit "off" or having a rough few days or so!

Have I confused you yet? Here's the reason. We are often… no… we are USUALLY the last ones to notice that something is a bit off or that we're just not ourselves. We may know that we've had a few not-so-good days, but what we usually don't notice is that it's medicinally-related or that the tiredness we've felt or the extra hour or two of sleep we've needed lately is a symptom of depression. Or that the fidgeting we've done all week and the slight pain in our chest is anxiety. Or that the annoying music we've been hearing outside isn't really music at all but a sign of impending psychosis. Nope. We tend not to notice these things at all. We don't put two and two together like that nearly as quickly as others do because to us, these things have become pretty normal.

My support system consists of my husband, my mother, and three close friends who have known me very, very well for a long time. Although my husband is the only one who sees me and interacts with me on a daily basis, I talk to my mom on the phone about twice a week, and I communicate with these friends often, both through social media, and on the phone, and we see each other occasionally. They know all about my history, and they wouldn't hesitate to tell me if they thought something were a bit "off." My mother, of course, has known me my entire life, and she well knows when I'm not myself, although she's learned that she has to be a bit delicate with me when suggesting that since I usually don't take it well coming from her, given our history together.

And now we get to my husband. He's always the first to notice when I'm not quite being myself and maybe, just maybe, it's time for a small tweak of the meds. I'll confess that it used to make me terribly angry when he would suggest that perhaps I needed an adjustment, but I now know that my anger was due to the fact that I couldn't figure it out for myself first. Of course, I should have been grateful. After all, two or three days later I always came around to agreeing with him, as if the whole thing were my idea in the first place. What he was trying to do was to save me from the complete overhaul that requires a hospitalization!

Once I made the decision that I was not going to do another inpatient hospitalization, I decided that it would behoove me to try to listen to him, even if I didn't want to. Oh, there were still times when I told him he was full of shit and that there was nothing at all wrong with me and nothing at all wrong with my medication, but I always came around. I'm happy to report now that I'm almost as quick at spotting the "off" days as he is—almost. But that has taken nearly ten years since I made that decision, nearly twenty years of being married, and nearly thirty years of having this diagnosis. Granted, I'm stubborn as a mule and probably could have reached this point much, much sooner had I wanted to, so don't expect to be able to do it overnight either!

Now… let's talk about what to look for in this support system.

Here are my suggestions:

1. If at all possible, I would include at least one family member with whom you interact on a daily basis. This could be a spouse, a parent, or a sibling. I do not recommend that you

ask one of your children to be part of your support system unless all of these three criteria are met:

    A. Your child is at least 30 years old and has a separate residence

    B. Your child was never traumatized in any way as a result of your mental illness

    C. Your child is not the only family member who is part of your support system

Believe it or not, there are some very concrete reasons for this. First, you don't want to put someone (anyone) who isn't pretty darned mature into the position of being part of your support system. I chose the age of 30 because in the vast majority of cases, by the time someone is 30 years old, he or she is independent, self-supporting, and understands what "adulting" is all about. Also, people in their thirties typically aren't still trying to live out their college years like people in their twenties often are. I know that I didn't really have much of a clue about life until I was close to thirty, and neither did most of the people I know, so that's a good age at which to formally declare someone an adult.

Also, even if your child is past the age of 30, if your mental illness caused him or her a great deal of trauma that is still unresolved, you do not want to ask this child to be part of your support system, and the simple reason is that he or she simply will not be able to view your ups and downs objectively. There will just be too much leftover baggage crowding the view. I'm not saying you're at fault or did anything wrong on purpose. We both know that when our illness takes over, we don't act like our normal selves, but children and teens don't understand that, and this trauma usually seeps right on into adulthood. There's no sense in further risking hurting your child by asking him or her to take on this responsibility—even if your child willingly offers to do it. This is a case where you need to politely decline.

Finally, if asking your child—whom let's say, is age 30 or above and whom wasn't traumatized in any way, shape, or form by your illness—will result in this child being the ONLY family member who is a part of your support system, you still don't want to do it. Now… if you add in a sibling or a spouse, that's fine, but including only a child (who meets the criteria) isn't a good idea. Again, relationships between parents and children tend to be a bit more delicate than those between you and your spouse or you and your siblings. They can also go wonky at times, often with no warning, so if you ask a child to be part of your system, be sure also to ask another family member, as well.

Once you have a family member (or two) in place, you'll want to add a few close friends. Remember that these friends should know you well and should know your mental health history. You don't want to have to explain this history to them at the time you ask them to be part of your support system. That's kind of awkward. In addition, these friends should be people with whom you are in communication on a regular basis. As much as you adored your best friend from high school, if it's been thirty years since you've seen each other, she's probably not the right person to ask.

You also want to make sure that you don't ask someone who has a real stigma about mental illness. Believe it or not (and I'm betting you'll have no trouble at all believing this), there are people out there who truly believe that depression is all "in your mind" and that if you just got out of bed and tried harder, you would be perfectly okay. (Can you believe???) There are also people who believe mental illness is a character defect or a personal weakness and can't imagine why you would need to take medicine for something such as that. I personally say, "To hell with these people. I don't need them in my life." But more about that later…

So... you've approached a few friends, and three have been happy to comply, but one just doesn't feel comfortable. No big deal. Just blow it off. Seriously. She probably doesn't understand enough about your illness and doesn't want to admit it. She also probably thinks that if you had an "off" few days or a week, she'd be personally responsible for making decisions for you or for "putting you away." You can tell her that's not true until you're blue in the face, but those words would probably fall on deaf ears. Just let it go. It doesn't mean she's not your friend.

What do you tell people about their "jobs" as people in your support system? Here's what I told my people:

"I'm not asking you to be my keeper or my watcher, and I'm not asking you to take responsibility for me in any way. All I'm asking you to do is to tell me if you see me acting a bit differently, strangely, or like I'm just not quite myself. That may mean that my medicine isn't working quite as well as it should, or it could mean nothing at all. I'm the last person to see these behavioral changes, so I'm asking you to be the eyes that see the changes first. The objective is to help me keep things on an even keel BEFORE a crisis occurs so I can avoid hospital visits and emergency trips to the psychiatrist. Sometimes all I need is a very small dosage change with one of my meds or even a change to a new drug. If we can work together on this, I can avoid the bad times and live a much happier, healthier life."

And that's all there is to it.

Now that we've formed our support system, we have to remember to USE IT.

When a member of your team tells you that you're not being "yourself," your job is to LISTEN. I protested for a very long time when my mom or my husband told me this, and it ended up costing me precious time that I could've used to get some help before things got worse. That was my fault. If you listen to these people and really stop to take note, you'll discover that 99% of the time, THEY'RE RIGHT. Does that mean that each time you're having an "off" day, you need a medicine change? No. Absolutely not. But several "off days" together and a few other strange things going on at the same time probably do mean that. One "off day" probably means you didn't sleep so well last night or have something on your mind. An "off week" is often something else entirely.

You'll learn to listen to your body. And with any luck, you'll also learn to listen to those in your support system. Once you learn to do both, you'll find that you can spot these "off" days very quickly and can get the help you need before the people outside your support system know that anything at all is wrong. Now THAT's taking charge of your illness!

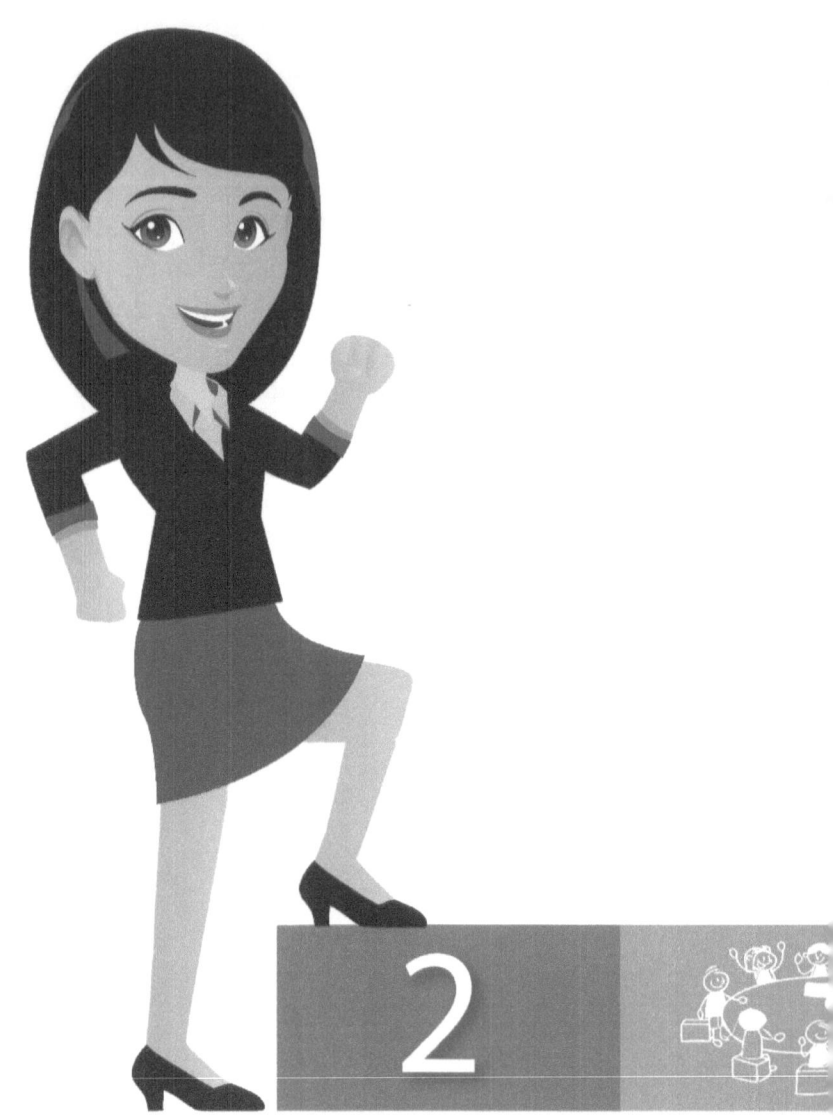

CHAPTER 9

Step 3: Practicing Daily Self Care

This step may sound to some people like a "duh" and to others like a "why on earth would this be something that would keep me from going into crisis?" step, but trust me when I tell you that it is an absolutely essential part of staying both mentally and physically healthy. I can tell you from experience that this is of paramount importance in order to keep oneself from quickly sinking into crisis mode and requiring hospitalization.

Back between 2004 and 2006, when I was frequenting the inpatient psychiatric facilities—and by frequenting, I mean making twice-a-year, week-long trips there—I was NOT practicing daily self care. In fact, I dare say that I wasn't practicing any kind of self-anything at all. I wasn't sleeping well, eating right, exercising well (I was actually OVER-exercising, which is just as bad as not getting any kind of exercise, if not worse), and I was stressed out all the time. Oh—and did I mention that I had three small children, a marriage, a demanding career, and I was immersed full-time in a doctoral program that required me driving an hour and a half one way to attend classes three days a week after working all day? Looking back on it, that would probably make someone WITHOUT a mental illness frequent the psych hospital!

So… about self care.

There are basically four things we must do to practice daily self care. I will discuss them here one at a time.

First, we have to get adequate sleep each night. By each night, I mean *every single night*. It's not okay to get your seven or eight hours of required sleep two or three nights in a row and then try to get by on for hours the next night, and repeat that cycle all over again. No, we need to get our sleep EVERY night. And if that means seeing an early movie rather than a late movie with your spouse or telling your girlfriends that you're happy to go clubbing with them but that you'll be bringing your own car because you have to be home by midnight, then that's what it means. I'm dead serious about this!

My friends know that the only time I ever sacrifice sleep is when I have to get up at the crack of dawn to catch an early flight. And even then, I go to bed earlier than usual the night before. I may end up getting 6 or 6 1/2 hours of sleep instead of 7 1/2 or 8 (my body really requires a full 8 hours), but that is the only time—and I do mean the ONLY time—when I don't get my 8 hours! It's just that important that I practice self care so I don't face a mental health crisis, and sleep is a big part of that. My family knows this, my friends know it, and anyone who doesn't respect it doesn't deserve to hang with me in the first place. Period. It's just that simple.

Now I know that there are quite a large number of people with mental health issues who have a great deal of trouble sleeping. This is a fact, and I'm not so naive as to think it's not. My suggestion is to let your psychiatrist know about this. There are some great meds on the market that help with sleep. I personally don't like the prescription sleep medicines, as they make me have weird dreams and do strange things in the middle of the night, as well as making me feel very hungover the next day. I take an antidepressant that doesn't work so well as an antidepressant but is wonderful at inducing sleep. I take it about 30 minutes before I'm ready to fall asleep, and I sleep like a baby. When I wake up the next morning, I feel great. No strange dreams, no hangovers, no nothing. I've been taking it for years, and it's very inexpensive, even without insurance. But everyone is different, and we all react to medicines in different ways, so talk to your doctor. There is no reason that without a little help that you shouldn't be sleeping well each night.

But what if I have the opposite problem, you ask? What if all I want to do is sleep? That's another indicator that you need to talk to your doctor. You shouldn't be feeling like that either. That means you're either depressed on a clinical level (We don't always get depressed for a "reason." Clinical depression may start like that, but it's not like that afterward)or something you're taking has the side effect of making you very, very sleepy. This may mean that that particular drug is not the right one for you. You don't just have to "get used to it" and walk around like a zombie all day! That's not what medicine is for! Your medicine is supposed to make you feel better, not worse. So talk to your doctor.

Now… the second part of self care is making sure you're eating right. When I say eating right, I mean that you're eating at least three meals a day, and at regular intervals. I say "at least" three meals because some folks are grazers, meaning that some people prefer to eat more frequent, smaller meals throughout the day, adding up to five or six meals. But hear me on this: YOU MAY NOT SKIP MEALS! Allowing yourself to get too hungry on a regular basis can throw your psyche into crisis mode very quickly. Do I want you to pig out all the time? Certainly not. Maintain a healthy wait, and eat decent food. But be sure to eat something for breakfast, lunch, and dinner. And also be sure to have some protein with each meal, as it's protein that sustains you between meals. Avoid the fad diets where you "can't eat" certain foods or cut out particular food groups all together. For one thing, they're very dangerous and can have lasting ill effects, and for another, when you deprive your body of certain foods, you're also depriving your brain, and remember it's your brain that you want to keep healthy, so feed it well.

It's also important to remember to try to maintain a healthy weight. I realize that there are some meds out there that are going to cause you to put on a few pounds. Others will make you not so hungry. Work with your doctor to keep your weight as stable as possible. Your body works best when you are at the healthiest weight possible. If you need to gain weight, do it healthily, not by eating a ton of junk food. If you need to lose weight, again, do it in a healthy way. Do NOT do the fad diets. Again, this is a time when you can work with your health care team. Nobody is saying that you need to have a super model's body. You certainly don't. You just want to aim to be a reasonable size so you can avoid having other health risks such as diabetes, high blood pressure, high cholesterol, etc. We can't control having our mental health issues, but we can control these other things, so why not at least try, right? I recently lost almost 40 pounds using an easy-to-get product that a high school friend introduced me to and have good success keeping it off. Nothing faddish about it, and I didn't cut out any food groups doing it. There ARE things out there that can help! It's just a matter of finding them!

The third thing we need to do to practice self care—and I know many of you are going to balk at this word—is to get some exercise. Wait! Before you skip over reading this section, I am not saying that you need to join a gym and get into bodybuilding on a full time basis. Far from it. Of course, if you're the gym type and that's your thing, then by all means, go for it. I'm just saying that you need to spend some time moving your body. Find something that you like to do, and do it a few times a week. I actually enjoy getting into the gym and lifting weights, and afterward, spending a bit of time on the elliptical machine. I really, really like it. And would you believe, the thing I like most about it is going by myself, getting all into my head, and people-watching while I'm doing it? Really. That's my thing. Of course, right this minute it's killing me not to be able to go because I'm awaiting knee surgery, but I'll get back soon, and when I do, I'll be enjoying myself once again.

My daughter enjoys horseback riding. That's her thing. And believe me, she's not just sitting leisurely on the horse. She rides English and jumps those fences (not nearly as high as you see in the Olympics, but maybe one day!), so she's had her exercise—and so has Jack, the horse—by the time she's ridden 45 minutes or an hour with him! My point is this: Don't be a couch potato. Whether it's a walk around the block, a leisurely swim, a bike ride, a horse ride, or whatever, just MOVE three or four days a week. Exercise produces endorphins, which are as good or better than any antidepressant. If you don't believe me, ask your doctor, and he'll confirm it. You will feel so much better, and your stress levels will be decreased when you move.

Okay, I'm finished with the very small section on exercising. The fourth part of self care is reducing stress. I'm willing to bet that if you sleep well every night, eat three meals (that contain protein) per day, and get a bit of exercise three or four days a week, you're already going to be much, *much* less stressed than if you didn't do these things. However, learning to reduce the "other" stressors in our lives isn't as easily done as it is said. I well understand this.

I found, after I made the decision to make my mental health the most important thing in my life, that friends and family members were some of my biggest sources of stress. I bet you're wondering right now, "But what do you do about that? How do you get rid of THAT kind of stress???"

The answer is deceptively simple.

Cut them out of your life.

Yes, you read that correctly.

Cut them out of your life.

I'll say it one more time, just so we understand one another.

Cut the stressors out of your life.

I'm 100% serious about this. If excessive stress is what's causing your mental illness to rear its ugly head and send you into crisis mode, and your mental health crises are consistently landing you in the psychiatric ward at the hospital, then it's time to remove those stressors from your life. It's as simple as that.

But how on earth do I remove family members and people with whom I've been friends for years??? They'll hate me! They'll think I'm a horrible person!!! All my other friends will hate me! That whole side of the family will hate me!

First, let me tell you that no, "all" your friends and the "whole other side of the family" aren't going to "hate" you. Second, if you're being that stressed out by one or two people, chances are pretty good that you're not the only one who is being stressed by this person or these people. And third, it's really not your business what others think of you, just like it's really none of my business what others think of me (and I don't really care). It says nothing in my Laura Gray "contract" about having to be popular, and boy is that freeing!

Actually, when it comes down to cutting our "people stressors" out of our lives, it's pretty simple.

When it comes to these so-called "friends," you have two choices. You can either break up with them in person, telling them that the stress in your relationship is no good for your mental health, which is now the most important thing in your life, so you've made the decision to back away from him/her for awhile, and you sincerely hope that when things get more stable for both of you, you might be able to reconnect again one day, blah blah blah… Or, you can just stop accepting phone calls and invitations and ghost that person completely. It's entirely up to you. I've done it both ways, and I can tell you that in the end, I've been so relieved not to have that source of stress in my life that I've never had any desire to rekindle the relationship, so ghosting didn't make me feel guilty at all.

"Unfriending" relatives and in-laws is a little more difficult. If the person lives more than 50 miles away, it's a snap. Just don't accept invitations, and don't visit anymore. I've done that with a couple of toxic relatives, and I don't think they've even noticed. If the person is someone you can't avoid seeing, such as a close in-law who lives nearby or a parent or sibling, you need to have a bit more finesse.

I, myself, have a very close relative whom I decided a couple of years ago I could no longer be around because it just wasn't working for my mental health. This person was causing me a great deal of stress every time I saw him because he had his own mental health issues and refused to work on them. That wasn't my problem, necessarily, but his failure to address his own issues became my problem when he treated me like the same 13-year old child he had known 35 years ago. He didn't think I could make good decisions and told me as much, he was holding resentments against me from twenty plus years ago, and instead of working on his own issues, he preferred to sit around with others and talk about how sick he was and allow his issues to bleed out into the life of one of my other close family members. I simply had to get him out of my life.

So, I discussed this with my husband, who agreed that it had to happen, and even though I was scared to death to say anything, I told the "other" close family member what I needed to do. Fortunately, this person understood perfectly, and the two of us agreed that we would hang out and do things together, but not with the toxic family member in tow, and that when he was around, I would be cordial and polite, but wouldn't hang around to engage in any type of other activities. I'm happy to say that it has worked out quite well so far, and I am now no longer stressed by this person.

This is what I mean when I say that in order to preserve my mental health, I am willing to do just about anything necessary and cut out anything that isn't good for me—even if that means cutting certain people out of my life.

There you have it. When it comes to taking care of yourself, do these four things: get a good night's sleep every night, eat at least three meals a day, move your body often, and cut out the stressors in your life. These are the things that will put you on an even playing field with those who don't have a mental illness or other mental health issues. Heck—they may even put you ahead of the game!

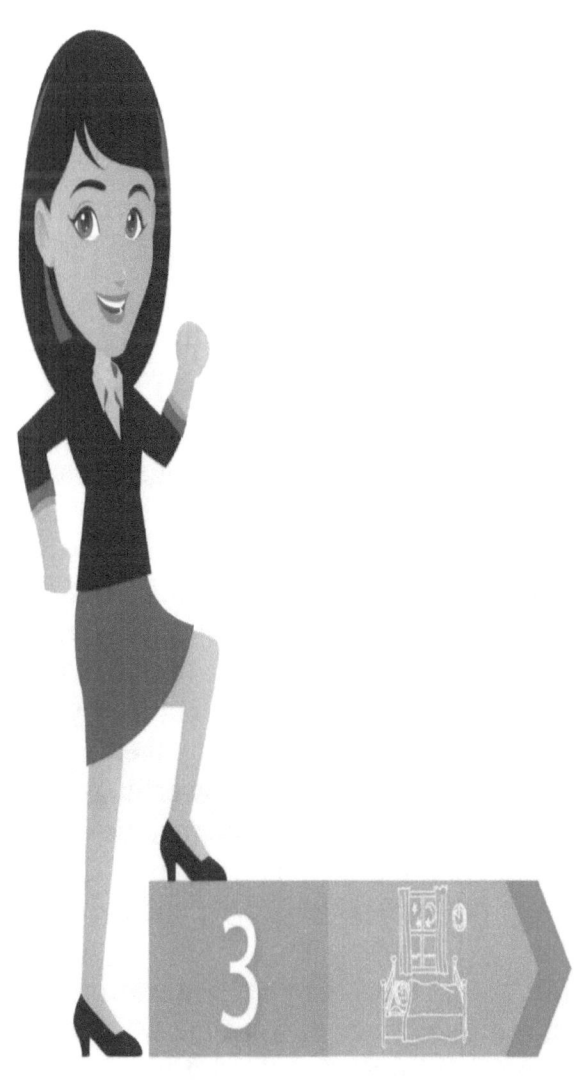

CHAPTER 10

Step 4: Living a Meaningful and Balanced Life

After I had my "break" and stopped working full time back in October of 2006, it took awhile to adjust to being at home, doing things during the daytime that I had normally always done after work or on the weekends, and ferrying the kids back and forth to and from all their various activities. I had never been a stay-at-home mom and wife, and I'll admit that the entire process felt downright weird. After a couple of years, though, I was completely in the groove, and by then I was feeling much better, so despite some very powerful guilt feelings of not contributing to the household income in a way that I thought I should, I had settled in and accepted—even relished, at times—my full-time roles of wife and mother.

At the same time, I still felt as if something was missing in my life. I knew that returning to work full-time wasn't an option, but I just didn't feel fulfilled. I wanted and needed something more, but I honestly had no idea what that "more" was. I just knew that getting the kids to school, going back to bed for two or three hours, and cooking and cleaning weren't doing it for me. It hit me one day that I had absolutely no goals in life. No goals for the day, the week, the year, and especially no goals for the long-term. That was a downright depressing feeling.

I decided I wanted to go back to school full time and complete my Ph.D. So, in late November of 2008 I put in my application to be re-admitted to the doctoral program I had abandoned two years earlier. By some miracle, the university and the department accepted me back, and in January 2009 I went back to school. Not only was I taking an online course, but I was also in the midst of my internship, which required me to be on-campus at a nearby community college three days a week. And as if that weren't enough, I decided that I'd work in my university's online learning lab 20 hours each week so my tuition would be paid and I'd receive a stipend. I dove right in, and there I was putting in a good 35-40 hours a week, having gone from zero hours per week the last two plus years.

Needless to say, that did not last long. By midterms, I was completely burned out and dropped out again. It had taken me two full months to realize I had taken on too much (which is not unusual for me) and couldn't handle it. My husband was disappointed in me, not for having quit again but for having bitten off more than I could chew in the first place, but I was even more disappointed in myself. To me, this represented yet another item in my long list of failures since early 2004 when I was spending two weeks a year in the hospital.

Several months later, though, I had my epiphany and realized that getting involved in something or taking something on didn't have to be at the level it had been years before. I decided that yes, I did want to finish my degree—but not right then. I did want to involve myself in something meaningful—but not everything in the world. I figured out that life was all about balance, and in order to stay healthy, I needed a balance of self-care and meaningful work in my life.

I started by volunteering. Early in 2010, my daughter tried out for and was placed on a competition cheerleading squad. Now, I don't know if you know about sports like competition cheerleading and travel sports, but they can take up a LOT of time, not only for the kids but for the parents as well. I was spending many, many hours at the gym where she practiced, so I decided to get involved in the parents' group and head up fund raising for the cheerleaders. (Competition and travel sports are also very expensive, so fund raising is a necessary part of it.) Lo and behold, I found out that I was good at it, and in a few short months' time, we had raised over $10,000 under my leadership.

Doing this gave me a big boost of confidence, and it took up enough of my time so that I wasn't sleeping constantly and watching Divorce Court and Dr. Phil on television every day. In addition, I was finally interacting with people with whom I had a shared interest. I had found something I enjoyed and that I was pretty successful with, and it gave my life the balance it needed for the remainder of the year.

Being the fund raiser chairman ran its course, and I eventually took on other small things such as substitute teaching at our children's school, getting involved in the PTA, and even doing some work for money here and there. I knew I was far, far from going back to work full time—even regularly on a part-time basis—but my life was much happier, and I was feeling better and better about myself all the time.

Finally, in the fall of 2011 I decided I was going to go back to school—this time online—and finish my Doctor of Philosophy degree once and for all. I began classes in January of 2012 in a 100% online program, and three years later, I graduated with my Ph.D. in instructional design for online learning with a perfect 4.0 average. Even before I completed the program, I had several job offers. This time, wisdom prevailed, and I took on two small part-time jobs. One was a contract position, and the other was as the facilitator of a couple of online courses. At first, I taught only two classes per semester, which was just enough to keep me engaged, keep me happy, and add some income to the household.

Over the past four years, my teaching duties have increased, and it is safe to say now that I work about 25-30 hours per week. However, all of my work is remote, and since I'm basically in charge of my time 98% of the time, I have the freedom to schedule other activities and appointments as I need and not be tied down to a 9-5 job. It's perfect for me. In addition, I started back attending professional conferences in 2015 and have presented dozens of times in the last three or four years. I've also published a bit, and I've gotten involved in a few professional organizations.

The key to all of this, though, was to start small and build things up as slowly as I could tolerate them. Finding balance in your life is not about taking on work and activities willy-nilly. It's about finding the one or two things outside of home life that are really meaningful to you and gauging your involvement according to your comfort level at the time. I do quite a bit these days, but there was a time not long ago when I positively could not have done everything I do now, and I also know that if I become burned out or feel that I've taken on too much, I can let something go, and it won't kill me or wreck my family's style of living.

So, how does one find something that is meaningful and adds balance to his or her life? The short answer is trial and error. You may have to try out a couple of things before you find something that sticks. A meaningful activity doesn't have to be work, either. It could be playing cards a couple of times a week with a group of friends or working on motorcycles with your buddy or your teenager. If you absolutely need to work and can't do without the income, look for something that isn't stressful and that you have control over. There are thousands upon thousands of legitimate work-from-home jobs that you can do online, many at a time of day when you are comfortable.

If you want to do volunteer work, there are also hundreds of organizations where you can volunteer right from the comfort of your home. Having the world at our fingertips via the Internet has been a godsend to many people with mental health issues who cannot or who don't want to go back to a "regular" type of job.

When you do find that your life has balance and meaning, you'll see that there are three things at work. First, you'll realize that you're practicing self-care on a daily basis and not sacrificing your sleep, meal time, or relationships for other things. Second, you'll find yourself looking forward to participating in whatever activities or work you've found, and that doing these things doesn't cause stress in your life. Finally, you will see that your confidence level has risen significantly, which, in turn, has led to an overall sense of well-being, and you will notice that you still have adequate free time in which to "chill out" and spend time with family and friends. You'll just smile more!

Finding balance and meaning in our lives is the key to staying healthy and having a sense of personal fulfillment. It gives us a reason to wake up in the mornings, as well as a reason to keep going on in those darker days when we begin to have intrusive thoughts or doubts about our abilities as humans. It takes away the stigma of being someone with a mental illness and replaces it with a sense that we're normal people doing normal things in a normal way—which we are—make no mistake about that. In short, it makes us better people.

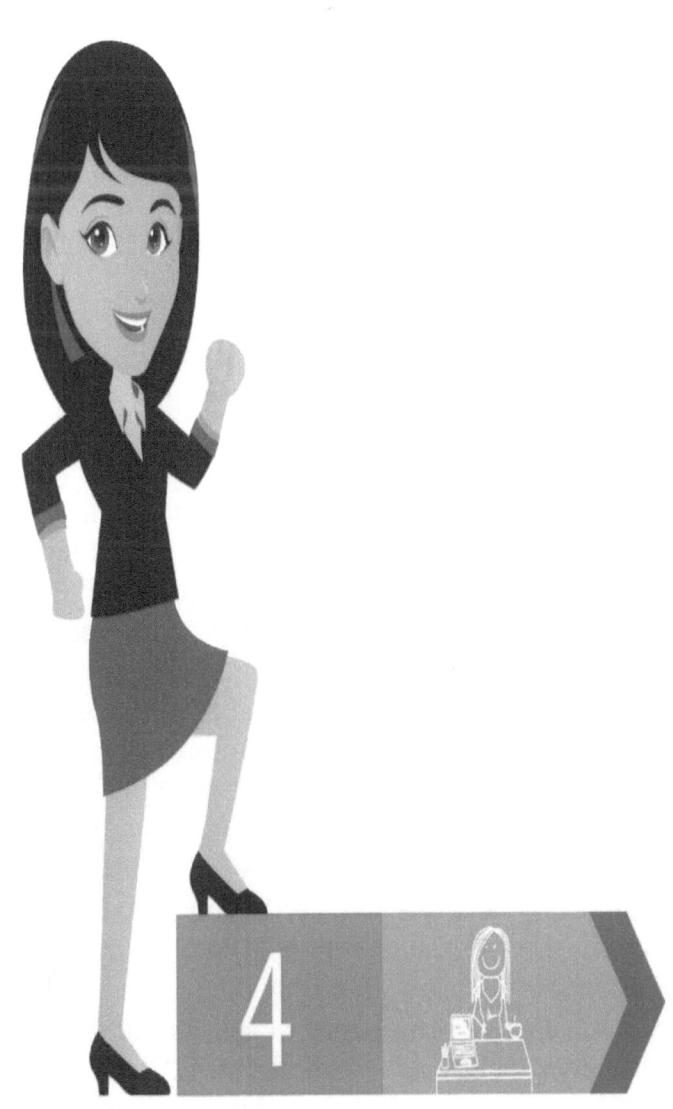

CHAPTER 11

Step 5: Advocating for Yourself and Others

Once you've got the first four steps down pat, you're going to find that you're really enjoying your new life. By then, not only will you have accepted your diagnosis, but you will also have put together a health care team that works for you, found a close-knit support system that watches your back, practiced daily self care until it becomes a habit, and found meaningful things to fill your life with. Wow! That's quite an accomplishment! So where do you go from here?

The fifth and final step to living your very best life is to get involved in advocacy, and this starts with yourself. For me, this involved becoming comfortable with talking about my mental illness and letting others know about my diagnoses and my experiences. Like I said a few chapters back, I used to be completely ashamed of having a mental illness. Because society has traditionally placed such a stigma on the mentally ill, I chose to buy into that stigmatization and kept my illness in the proverbial closet, so to speak. I was afraid that if others knew this about me that they either wouldn't like me or would somehow think less of me as a person.

What I have come to realize over the last several years is that if people can't accept that I have this illness and that there are certain things I HAVE to do in order to stay healthy, then I don't really want them in my life anyway. That may sound harsh, but it's true. I recently had an issue where I was told that I didn't need to be a member of a certain organization due to my illness. (Yes, this really happened, and unfortunately, it still sometimes happens. Sad, but true.) At first I was very hurt and very upset, but after I slept on it—which is a good idea when you're dealing with an upsetting situation that you can't control—I realized a couple of things. For one, it occurred to me that the people in this group were not the people with whom I wanted to spend time and devote my energy. Not at all. And second, it gave me even more resolve to stand up for myself and for my illness in order to erase the stigma and fear that some people still carry.

This brings us to advocating for oneself. Ultimately, if you don't stand up for your illness and advocate for yourself, you can't count on anyone else to advocate for you. Now… I'm not speaking to those who have been recently diagnosed and maybe haven't gotten a handle on their situation or haven't yet found medication that alleviates their symptoms. I'm speaking to those who have followed the first four steps outlined in this book and have ended up on Step Five. Let me be clear here: If you are still struggling, you're not "there" just yet. But, if you have worked successfully through the first four steps, you're definitely ready to step up to the plate and advocate for yourself and others!

So… how do you do that, exactly? Advocating can come in many forms. If you've kept your illness in the closet from certain friends and family members, now is the time to be honest and tell them about your diagnosis and your transformation. Show them how far you've come. Tell them that you are *not* the sum total of your illness and that you *are* taking good care of your brain. In other words, the best example of self-advocacy is to let others see you living your best life!

Another way to advocate for yourself (and help others at the same time) is to get involved with a local mental health association. NAMI (National Alliance for the Mentally Ill) has numerous chapters all over the country, and they actually seek out people who have done very well in spite of their diagnoses to speak to certain groups in order to help reduce the stigma of mental illness and to show others that mental health issues are nothing to be afraid of. If you have a spouse or close family member who has been with you every step of the way, NAMI chapters also have family groups that are run by and for family members of those with mental illness. These groups offer education and support, and they're also a wonderful way to meet others who truly understand the situation. NAMI can be found online at https://www.nami.org. Membership can be either free or paid, depending on your circumstances and your desires, and in my humble opinion, what you get in return is totally worth it.

Another good organization where you can practice your advocacy skills is MHA (Mental Health America). This organization provides screening for mental health disorders and also helps connect people with psychiatrists, psychiatric nurse practitioners, and therapists. In addition, MHA does fantastic work within the communities where their chapters are located. They serve meals to those (with mental illnesses) in need, provide support groups and fellowship opportunities, and also work with local homeless people who are suffering from mental health disorders. This is a true grass-roots organization that accomplishes the vast majority of its goals with help from volunteers. If you live near an area where MHA functions, working with this group will not only help you to advocate for yourself, but it will also help a hundred-fold in terms of assisting those who are not yet well enough to advocate for themselves. MHA can be found online at https://www.mentalhealthamerica.net.

Should your diagnosis be that of depression, Bipolar I, Bipolar II, or Schizoaffective Disorder (Bipolar's close first cousin), DBSA, or the Depression and Bipolar Support Alliance, is a great group to get involved in. Again, this is a nationally-known group with chapters all across the country, and their mission is to provide education, support, and advocacy for both consumers and family members. There are multiple ways to get involved with DBSA and help others, as well as yourself. DBSA can be found at https://https://secure2.convio.net/dabsa/site/SPageServer/?pagename=home, or you can simply Google "depression and bipolar support alliance" online, and you will be directed to the site. There are numerous DBSA in-person and online chapters throughout the United States.

The other really neat thing about DBSA is that they sponsor peer support trainings so that those who have "been there, done that" and want to give back to the community can become certified peer support specialists. Obtaining this certification requires a full week (40 hours) of training, plus an online exam. However, the rewards can be tremendous. If you find that you're doing well and want to help others, becoming a certified peer support specialist is a wonderful thing to do!

And last (but certainly not least!), there is the Anxiety and Depression Association of America (ADAA). This is another national group that seeks to help, educate, and advocate for those with all forms of anxiety (generalized anxiety disorder, hoarding, agoraphobia, social anxiety, OCD, body dysmorphic disorder, PTSD, and the like) and depressive (seasonal affective disorder, bipolar disorder, and clinical depression) disorders. Again, they have support groups all over the country, both in-person and online, and the structure is peers helping peers. Their online address is https://adaa.org.

Of course, if you're an avid social media user, you may find that certain individuals "out there" have taken it upon themselves to begin groups of their own. I'll put in a shameless plug for my group right now. I run a Facebook group call Stable, Strong, and Stigma-Free. Not a support group, this is a group for anyone who has dealt with a mental health issue and wants to receive education and coaching on exactly how to go about living their very best lives. I actually got the idea back when I started writing this book. I feel so strongly about the Five-Step Program that I want to share it with as many people as I possibly can. So... if you're so inclined, come see me at https://www.facebook.com/groups/stablestrongstigmafree. My program is a piggy-back off of this book. I work personally with those who want not only to learn the Five Steps but also want to fully incorporate them into their lives. And... if you mention that you've read this book when you come to the group, I'll give you a discount on my services! Promise!

In addition to the well-known groups that are out there, finding ways to advocate for yourself and others can be as simple as speaking to your local Parent/Teacher group on mental health issues and sharing some of your own story. It can also be volunteering at a homeless shelter, as we know that many who are homeless suffer from some kind of mental health disorder. Whatever you decide to do, and however large a scale you decide to do it, remember that this step is just as important as the others—if not moreso. After all, if we don't advocate for ourselves and others, nobody else will.

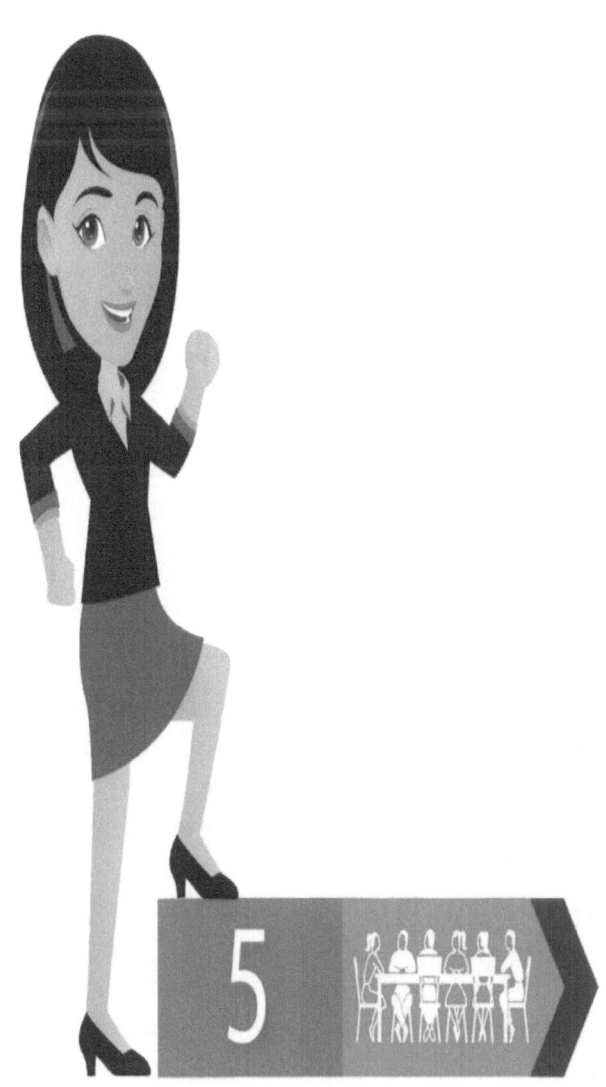

CHAPTER 12

Putting it All Together and Living the Life You've Always Wanted

Well… now that you have a good understanding of THE 5-Step Plan, how do you go about getting it done and putting it all together?

Excellent question.

I can't tell you exactly what your life is going to look like after you commit yourself to the Plan and work the steps, but I can assure you—100%—that it's going to be WAY better than it was before you started! (Promise!). Since everyone's life is different, and we all function as individuals, I can only tell you what my life looks like now that I've put these five steps into practice.

First, I have fully accepted that my illness is a part of me—but doesn't define me—and, as such, I've put together a team of wonderful health-care professionals who are totally committed (as long as I am) to seeing that I take the right medications in the right dosages and that I am constantly and consistently working on my issues in therapy. I'll admit, it's not always rainbows and unicorns every time I see my psychiatrist or therapist. In fact, my therapist frequently tells me, "Laura, you're full of shit." But that's okay because that's what I need to hear when I start obsessing about why I have a hater on Facebook who likes to post in my Stable, Strong, and Stigma-Free group or why I'm so obsessed about having enough money to live on (but that's another story for another time, and after all, it is MY issue). All in all, though, I know that my psychiatrist and therapist both have my best interest at heart, as does my family practice doctor, and they are willing to communicate with one another in order to see that I receive the best care possible.

Second, I can tell you that my support system is there to see to it that I'm running on an even keel most of the time. Again, it's not always fun and games with these people either. I certainly don't like it when my mom ever so gently indicates that I'm being unreasonable (even if she's right), but I do make a point to stop and take a closer look at my reactions and my motives when she does point something out, just as I do when my husband says something to me—which, by the way, is much more frequently since I live about 1000 miles from my mother. And, of course, the friends in my support system check on me when they haven't heard from me in awhile and are the first to ask if everything's okay when I make cryptic posts on social media.

Gladly, these things don't happen very often, but when they do, I know I've got people who keep an eye on me and who are concerned for my well-being when I'm not quite myself. (And when I say "myself," I mean my happy, stable self, or Dr. Jekyll, as my husband likes to call it, rather than the deranged Mr. Hyde.)

Third, I have found that it's not difficult at all to live the life I want while taking care of myself on a daily basis. I have a pretty normal routine for someone who still has a kid in school and who works from home. I wake up around 7:00 each morning to make sure The Spawn (my daughter) is awake, I pore over Facebook for awhile, and before 8:00 I'm in the shower, starting to get ready for the day. I usually begin my work day around 10:00 a.m. and try to wind things down between 5:00 and 6:00 p.m., but I do a great deal of loafing in-between, as I still have difficulty with focusing for long periods of time. If I have somewhere to be during the day or an errand to run, I can usually get away and take care of it.

By 6:00, everyone in the house is usually in for the evening, and we cook dinner (or order out), and my husband and I like to pick up on whichever show we're currently watching on Netflix or Hulu. By about 9:00 p.m., I'm usually pretty tired, so I get in the bed, and again, wind down with a little social media and reading a few chapters of one of the many non-fiction books I have on my Kindle. (In case you're wondering, I generally don't read fiction. I like to read about true crime, religion and philosophy, and trivia. I realize it's a strange mix, but hey—nobody ever said I wasn't a little strange.) Then, by 10:00 or 10:30, it's lights out for me.

On the weekends, I usually have a bit of work to do so I can get ready for the upcoming week, but I generally like to relax with the family, shop, eat out somewhere new, or hang out with friends doing low-key things. My husband and I also enjoy traveling whenever we can, so we try to do that three or four times a year (Of course, the work comes with me, except for the weeks before and after Christmas when I am officially "off.")

Fourth, and I think this ties into what I've already said, I have found enjoyable and meaningful things to occupy my time and keep my life in balance. I absolutely love my work as a remote university professor, and I also belong to a couple of women's business organizations. In addition, I make sure that two or three times a month, I get together with friends. Of course, my husband and I also enjoy our date nights once or twice a month, and he is really good about keeping tabs on how much I'm working to make sure that I'm not over-doing it. (I may have mentioned earlier that I have a tendency to be kind of a workaholic.)

Finally, I derive immense joy from my involvement in mental health organizations and initiatives. I really want to help those who are at a crossroads with their mental health issues… those who KNOW there's a better way to a better life out there, but who just haven't found a way to make it work yet. For the past several years, I've wanted to find a way to personally help people find a way to a new life, which is what inspired me to create Stable, Strong, and Stigma-Free. I'm happy to report that this group is growing by leaps and bounds, and I see nothing but good things ahead!

So, in a rather large nutshell, that's what my life looks like, having put all of these steps in action. Do I have bad days? Certainly. Do I need the occasional med tweak or even a med change? Yes. In fact, over the last year and a half, I've had more medication changes than I have in the last ten years combined. It happens to all of us. But I haven't even come close to needing hospitalization or a complete "overhaul," and I count that as a HUGE win every day.

Again, I can't say what's out there for you or what your new life will look like, but I'd really and truly love to know once you get there. My e-mail address is on the back cover of this book, so be sure to write and tell me about your journey and your successes. I count those as big wins, too!

That's all for now. My plan now is to take a couple of months off from writing and then to begin the second in this series of books, which will be a book devoted entirely to Step 1 of THE 5-Step Plan. In the meantime, I sincerely wish you the best, and there's nothing I want more than for you to take charge of your diagnosis and life a happy, balanced life!

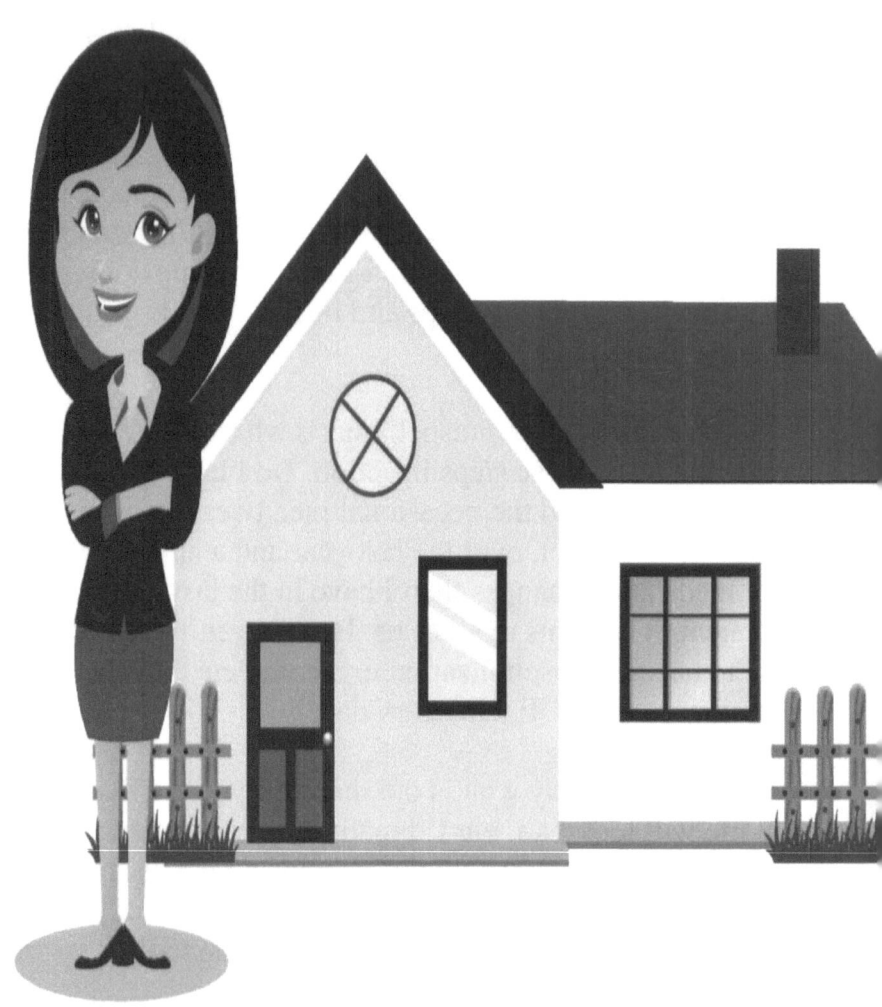

Contacting the Author

Dr. Gray is available for speaking engagements, workshops, coaching, and retreats at your location, tailored specifically to your personal needs or to your group's needs.

You may reach her by joining the Stable, Strong, and Stigma-Free Facebook Group at https://www.facebooko.com/groups/stablestrongstigmafree, or you may e-mail her at stablestrongandstigmafree@gmail.com.

www.ingramcontent.com/pod-product-compliance
Lightning Source LLC
Chambersburg PA
CBHW022128170526
45157CB00004B/1786